MASTER YOUR CHRONIC PAIN

A Practical Guide

Nicola Sherlock

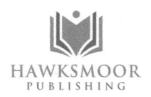

HAWKSMOOR
PUBLISHING

First published 2021 by Hawksmoor Publishing

Kemp House, 152-160 City Rd, London, EC1V 2NX

www.hawksmoorpublishing.com

ISBN: 978-1-914066-10-8

To Shane and Mark

For telling me that I should and that I could.

I first thought about writing this book while chatting to my brother at my kitchen table. As I once again sit here at my table, now with a completed book, I am conscious that so many people helped me in my journey from contemplation to completion. There are a few people that I would like to give special thanks to:

To my fantastic pain team colleagues – Dr Jones, Dr McConaghy, Dr McMullan, Dr Sobocinski, Michelle McGeown, Emma Moley, Patrick O'Farrell, Briege McAnerney, Maggie McCartan, Patricia McCrystal, Blinne McGee, Nicola Mawhinney, Heather Stafford and Brona Nugent. Your warmth and support over the years means so much to me. You have generously shared your expertise and knowledge, and you have been great fun to be around – thank you.

To Ellen Pietersen – thank you for your editing of my first draft and for encouraging me along the way.

To James Lumsden-Cook – for believing in this book.

To Mum and Dad – for passing on your values of compassion and perseverance.

To Kieran, Gary, Paul, Ryan and Mark – your achievements inspire me every day.

To Shane – for always believing in me.

To Jack, Alex, and Max. Thank you for learning to cook and allowing me the time to write.

Finally, I want to thank my patients. You have trusted me and opened your hearts to me. Thank you for allowing me to walk with you for a while.

Nicola

Table of Contents

PROLOGUE

*The wound is the place where
the light enters you.*
Rumi

I thought that I had finished this book, but then something happened in my life that led me to write this prologue. The week that I finished the first draft of the book, I developed sciatica.

Initially, it developed as a feeling of pins and needles in my right leg, then over a period of a couple of weeks, it got more painful. I took a few days off work and subsequently returned feeling much better.

About a week after my return to work, however, the sciatica returned with a vengeance. I experienced rip-roaring leg pain. The pain was worse when I sat down, and if I had to sit for more than a few minutes, it became almost unbearable. I could barely walk and struggled to find a comfortable lying position. I couldn't believe that this had happened to me out of the blue! I was fit and healthy, working out in the gym five or six times a week. Overnight, I became someone who could barely walk; someone who couldn't sit and couldn't work.

For months there was little improvement, but gradually my pain began to improve. As I write this, my sciatica has significantly improved and I have recently returned to work, even though the pain has still not resolved. I am hopeful that I am on the road to recovery. I don't know what that recovery will look like; I am unsure whether I will be pain-free or whether I – like you – will have to learn to live with pain. Before I finally finished this book, I wanted to reflect a little bit about my experience of living with pain; pain that was often intense, over a period of months.

I have learned that fear of movement is a very real thing! I have spent most of my professional life working in a persistent pain service, and I know that remaining active is an important part of recovering and living with pain. I also know that after I developed my pain, whenever I was active, my mind *screamed* at me to stop it.

My physiotherapist encouraged me to go for short walks, walks of around 10 minutes duration if I could manage it. I understood the rationale behind this, I have read the research literature on activity, and I had written the book on it! But still, my mind tried to persuade me that every painful step was too difficult, and that my body was not meant to move when I was in this much pain. I had to work hard to become an observer of my mind. I had to remind myself – again and again – that my mind may not always provide the most helpful advice. I had to remember that even though my slow, shuffling walks were painful, they would ultimately help my recovery.

It is difficult to accept that you cannot make the pain go away. I have written about acceptance and how the struggle against unwanted thoughts, emotions, and physical sensations can increase your suffering. I knew that it would be better for me if I could accept my situation, but I found this challenging. It was hard to accept that I was in pain and that I had to take some time out from work. I hadn't time to be off work! Initially, I thought that I could just push through the pain, and I adopted that "No Pain, No Gain" mentality that I caution against later in this book. This approach didn't last long. I quickly learned that it wasn't going to work and that I needed to accept that pain was part of my life, that I couldn't make it disappear, and (surprise, surprise) I had to learn to manage it!

It is hard to live in the present. For a number of years, I have been practising mindfulness meditation and trying to be more mindful and present in my everyday activities. When my sciatica was really bad, when nothing seemed to be helping it, I struggled to live in the present, even for short periods of time. My mind was constantly jumping to the future, telling me stories about how I would never be able to walk properly again, how I would never be able to go back to the gym, how I would not be able to do my job again due to my inability to sit for more than a couple of minutes, and on and on and on. I was grateful for my ability to recognise that my mind was telling me stories and that I could choose to listen to these stories (and take on board the dire predictions), *or* I could choose to be present, to notice where I was – what I could see, smell, touch, feel.

I have also learned that pacing is a challenge! Over the years, I had noticed many patients struggling with pacing activity. When it became necessary for me to pace my activity, I also struggled. It was very difficult to put the iron down when only a few more items needed ironing. It was very hard not to keep pushing on when I had only spent 10 minutes tidying a room. I learned the hard way that pacing *does* work and that it is better to do less, more often, than to try to push through the pain all the time and pay the price with a real spike in pain levels. I also learned to accept that the pace at which I did things was much slower than I would have liked.

I discovered how quickly and easily pain can come to define you. My pain was the first thing that friends and family asked about when they phoned me or met me face to face. Even strangers in a shop asked about my pain; seeing my limping gait, they wondered if I had hurt my ankle. I knew that they were asking about it out of concern, but it was as if everything else in my life had diminished – it was all about the pain. This gave me an insight into how quickly pain can take over your life.

I engaged in a lot of self-reflection. I tried to see if there were any positives in a situation that seemed entirely negative. I learned that this experience of living with pain provided me with the opportunity to be a bit more compassionate with myself, to slow down and take time for the relaxation that my body had been crying out for. *I came to see that the wound is the place where the light enters you.*

Finally, experiencing this pain confirmed what I have always known. Living with pain is far from easy and that getting up in pain every day, and going to bed in pain every night, can be draining. However, while I have only lived with pain for a few months, my experience has confirmed to me that there are things we can do to make our lives better and that it is possible to live a life of meaning, even if that life is lived in pain.

INTRODUCTION

Chronic or persistent pain is a big problem. A vast number of people live with pain on a daily basis. It has been estimated that chronic pain affects almost 10 million Britons and 50 million Americans of all ages. In turn, the treatment of back pain alone costs the British Exchequer in the region of £5 billion per annum. Many people living with pain are not able to work and are not even covered by this figure. However, as a Pain Psychologist, I am less interested in the economic cost of pain and more interested in the personal cost, which can be devastating.

If you are living with chronic pain, your pain may be a hidden problem. Even if you use a crutch, wheelchair, or another device to help with mobility, it is probably not obvious to others that you are in pain. You may end up living a secret life of pain. Yes, your close family and friends may know about your pain, but they may struggle to understand what experiencing pain on a daily basis is really like. And that can feel very lonely.

It can be hard to be hopeful about the future when you live in pain every day. You go to your GP or doctor and might have been prescribed medication, but those "pain killers" don't kill your pain. It can be very hard to understand why the medical profession – who can transplant a heart or perform delicate surgery on newborns – cannot cure your pain. Many people that I have worked with had initially been quite hopeful when they first developed their pain. They attended their GP with the expectation that medication would cure their problems. Months down the line, hope started to fade and – for some – despair had begun to set in.

Chronic pain can impact many aspects of life. Here are some ways that pain may have affected your life:

- **Activity levels** – you may have become much less active over time.

- **Struggle to do everyday tasks** – you may struggle to carry out some everyday tasks; tasks that you used to do without a thought. For example, you may now struggle to vacuum your home, put on your socks and shoes, or do the gardening. These struggles may leave you feeling very frustrated.

- **Working life** – you may have had to give up work due to pain. If you have been able to remain in work, you may have had to reduce your hours, take periods of sick leave, and you may not have progressed with your career as quickly as you had planned.

- **Financial worries** – you may have financial concerns due to a reduced income or your inability to work.

- **Anxiety** – you may notice that you are worrying more about life and the future.

- **Low mood** – you may feel down or depressed.

- **Social life** – you may not socialise as often.

- **Hobbies and interests** – you may have let go of formally enjoyed hobbies, especially those of an active nature. You may have lost interest in hobbies.

- **Sleep** – you may be unable to sleep and feel constantly fatigued.

- **Medication** – you may have to take medication on a frequent or daily basis. You might have to cope with the unpleasant side effects of your medication, like constipation and sedation.

- **Irritability and anger** – you may feel irritable and angry more often, and you may find that you are 'taking it out' on your nearest and dearest family and friends.

- **Relationship difficulties** – you may notice that some of your relationships have deteriorated, perhaps due in part to your irritability and feelings of frustration.

- **Difficulties with intimate relationships** – you may experience low libido or sexual difficulties. These can be related to your pain, low mood, and/or side effects of pain medication.

- **Guilt** – You may feel guilty about the change in role that you have experienced as a result of your pain. Perhaps you can no longer provide financially for yourself and your family in the way you did before you developed your pain. Maybe you can no longer go swimming with your children or care for your grandchildren. You might feel guilty that you are letting your family down.

- **Withdrawal** – you may notice that you have become more withdrawn from others, including family and friends. Perhaps you are not seeing friends as often as you did before, or perhaps you are isolating yourself from family members.

- **Troublesome thoughts** – you may experience upsetting thoughts that cause you to feel bad. You may experience thoughts like "I am useless" or "I should be able to manage this pain."

- **Not feeling as confident** – you may have noticed that you are not as confident as you were before you developed your pain.

- **Hopelessness** – you may feel hopeless about the future.

Why Should You Read This Book?

I have spent twenty years working in a pain service in the NHS. Over the years, I have met with many thousands of patients who have shared their stories with me. I have used the research that has been carried out in the chronic pain field to help those people manage their pain and live better lives. I believe that it is now time to share my clinical experience in this book to help you better live your life with pain.

Traditionally, we have relied on medicine to provide the answers to health problems, and over the years, the role of medication in pain management has been heavily emphasised. Medication and/or medical interventions may play an important role in the management of your pain.

I work very closely with my medical colleagues and fully appreciate the important role that they play in helping people manage their pain. But medication and/or medical interventions are only part of the picture.

I want you to imagine that you are a DIY enthusiast and you are given a brand-new toolbox as a Christmas present. You open the toolbox and see that it contains only one thing… a hammer. That hammer will be useful to you; you can now do a number of the DIY tasks on your list. But what about the other tasks that need other tools? How much more effective would you be if you have a toolbox that contained many different tools? Well, pain management is like that – it takes more than one tool to effectively manage pain. And whilst medicine offers one pain management tool, there is a whole world of other pain management tools available.

Since the 1960s, there has been an explosion of research in pain management, and we now have a much better understanding of how pain is perceived and experienced, and more importantly, how we can better manage pain.

My working life has been focused on using the research to give hope to people who live with chronic pain by providing them with the tools they can use to get their lives back.

Most patients that I have worked with have told me that their pain has had a detrimental impact on many areas of their life. *Very many* patients, though, have told me that their pain has had such a significant impact on them that they feel like the 'pause button' has been pressed on their lives since they developed their pain. Yes, they are still breathing, but they are merely existing or not living the rich and meaningful lives they used to. I know that it does not have to be like that! That can be hard to believe, I appreciate; when you live with daily pain, it can be difficult to believe that life can be good and meaningful even with pain. But my years of practice have taught me otherwise, and I want to share the knowledge and skills that I have learned, so that you can move forward with a meaningful, full life. So, let's get started!

HOW TO USE THIS BOOK

Chapters 1-14 in this book cover different pain management tools. I hope that by the end of this book, you will have the information you need to feel empowered to master your pain and improve your quality of life.

I think that it is best if you read this book in the order in which it is written. The chapters are designed to build upon the information that has been presented in previous chapters. If the chapter does not seem particularly relevant to you, at first glance, I would urge you to read it anyway, as I think that you are likely to find something that could benefit you in each chapter. Once you have read the book, you may decide to go back and focus on specific chapters or steps that seem particularly meaningful to your life.

It would be helpful to use a notebook or journal while reading the book as it contains several pen and paper exercises. To gain the most benefit from the book, you should complete all the exercises. Keeping all your notes in one place allows you to refer back to them easily.

I would also suggest that you consider asking close family members/friends to read this book. As the saying goes, 'no man (or woman) is an island', and it is important that you feel supported when you are making changes in your life. It can be hard for family and friends to understand your pain, the impact that it has on your life, and why it has persisted for so long. They may also feel frustrated or angry that nobody has been able to take away or cure your pain.

It may be hard for family and close friends to understand why you are changing aspects of your life (for example, why you are starting to put a few minutes aside each day to meditate); if your family and close friends can increase their understanding of your pain and the rationale for the changes that you are making in your life, they will be in a much better place to support and encourage you to move forward with your pain management journey.

CHAPTER 1: UNDERSTAND YOUR PAIN

> *The highest action a human being can attain is learning for understanding because to understand is to be free.*
>
> **Baruch Spinoza**

Chronic pain is difficult to understand. Why does it persist? Why did your friend's back pain resolve in a fortnight, whilst your pain carries on year after year? Why have you been given a diagnosis of Fibromyalgia when your blood tests show up nothing abnormal?

I believe that increasing your understanding about pain is one of the most important steps that you can take towards a better life. There is very good research evidence to suggest that if you understand your pain better, you will be able to manage it better. If you can manage it better, your quality of life will improve.

The Good News and the Bad News

I have some good news and some bad news about chronic pain. Let's start with the bad news and get that out of the way.

> ## There is no quick fix for chronic pain.

Many of you will know that already. Some of you may struggle to read that sentence. I can understand that. If you live with pain on a daily basis, it is completely normal to want a cure for that pain. If you are lucky enough to have the financial resources, you may have spent thousands of pounds looking for that cure. The very fact that you are reading this book suggests that you haven't found it yet. You may have found things that help with your pain. Many of my patients, for example, tell me that things like medication, reflexology, and acupuncture have helped their pain. But none of those pain relief options provides a cure or completely takes away their pain.

At the beginning of this book, I explained that I aim to provide you with tools to help you manage your pain. I used the term *manage* and not cure because there is no quick fix or cure for chronic pain. If I had that cure, I would pass it onto you in a heartbeat.

So that's the bad news out of the way. Now for the good news.

> **There are many, many things that you can do to help you manage your pain and improve your quality of life.**

When you read that sentence first, and particularly when you see the word *manage*, you may feel disappointed or angry. We are used to instant gratification. If I have a headache, I can take a couple of paracetamols and expect it to be gone within an hour. Why can't chronic pain be like that? Why is there nothing that can instantly take it away? I don't have the answers to those questions. It does not seem fair that some people have to live their life in pain.

But back to the good news – knowledge is power and if you can begin to understand your pain, you are taking the first important step in your journey to a better life.

Let's look at some of the terms used in the medical literature.

Acute Pain

All of us experience pain at a very young age. One of my earliest painful memories is falling, head first, off a bike and injuring my arm. Even at that young age, I knew that the pain would fade as my arm healed. What was the function of that pain? Well, it let me know that I should go to my mother to let her examine my arm, and if necessary, I knew that she would take me to the hospital for an x-ray. What would have happened if I had not felt that pain? I would have probably just dusted myself off and got on with my day. But what if I had a serious injury to my arm? What if I had broken my arm and not got it treated? This pain was useful pain (although it did not feel like it at the time!) because it alerted me to a problem that had to be dealt with.

> **Acute pain is a helpful alarm signal that enables us to get out of harm's way and protects our body as we heal. Therefore, the primary function of acute pain is to tell the body about injury and disease and to help us make decisions about what to do.**

There is a rare genetic condition, known as Congenital Insensitivity to Pain, that results in a person being unable to perceive pain. I bet that some of you would love to have that condition. Not unsurprisingly, it comes with a price – people who have this condition often die prematurely. For example, what happens if they develop appendicitis but have no pain? Their appendix could rupture, putting their lives at risk. This condition provides us with further evidence that pain can be useful and functional. We can conclude that although pain is unpleasant, it is a useful sensation to have.

The type of pain experienced by me after my fall from my bike is known as acute pain. Acute pain is short-lived and can last from a couple of seconds to around three months or until the stage at which we would expect healing to have been completed. Examples of acute pain conditions include toothache, bone fractures, and sprains. We know that acute pain usually responds well to medication. After acute pain has gone away, people can get on with life as normal.

Chronic or Persistent Pain

Chronic and persistent pain are both medical terms, and they essentially mean the same thing. When I started my career, chronic pain was the term that was most commonly used by clinicians to describe pain that went on for a long period of time. More recently, the term persistent pain is being used by clinicians, and I consider this to be a better term as it clearly describes the enduring nature of long-term pain. From here on, in this book, I will use the term persistent pain.

So, what is persistent pain? Well, the first important characteristic of persistent pain is associated with the duration of the pain. As the name suggests, this pain persists or carries on. How long does it carry on for? Unfortunately, it can continue for many years. It is not uncommon for me to see patients in my clinic who have had pain for more than 20 years.

Generally, in the scientific literature:

> **Chronic or persistent pain is regarded as pain that has persisted for more than three months or beyond the stage of expected tissue healing.**

The second (and I think most important) characteristic of persistent pain is that

> **It serves no useful purpose and is not an indication of new or further damage.**

So, let's look at the first part of that sentence. It serves no useful function. Unlike acute pain, it is of no benefit to us. If I took out a magic wand and got rid of your pain, I am sure that you could live a very normal life without it. In fact, I would guess that you would give me a lot of money to use that magic wand on your pain!

The second part of the sentence is a little harder to believe. Persistent pain is not an indication of new or further damage. When I tell my patients this, they often look at me in disbelief – surely Nicola does not know what she is talking about! I can easily appreciate how this is difficult to accept. As I said earlier, from a young age, we have learned about pain. By the time of our first birthday, we have experienced pain a number of times. For the vast majority of us, the pain that we have experienced in our earlier years has been acute pain, and it is not helpful to use acute pain as a gauge to understand persistent pain. Persistent pain is different from acute pain, and the characteristics associated with acute pain (falling off my bike) do not apply to persistent pain (back pain that has plagued somebody for years).

Let me tell you a little bit about the latest research in the field of persistent pain. But before we look at the research further, it is important to emphasise a very important research finding:

> **Persistent pain is 'real pain'.**
> **Even if you have not been given a**
> **definitive diagnosis for your pain.**

Persistent pain is as real as the pain that I felt during labour and is as real as the pain I felt last night when I burned my hand doing the ironing!

Unfortunately, it can be very difficult to find an exact physical cause for some people who have persistent pain. People can have really severe pain, but nothing shows up in x-rays or scans. To further add to the confusion, even if doctors can pinpoint physical changes on a scan or x-ray, it might be still impossible to say if this physical change is the cause of the pain. For example, a doctor can have scans belonging to two different patients. The patient who has no pain or very mild pain can have physical changes on their scan, while the patient who has severe pain may have nothing significant evident on their scan. This finding just serves to highlight how complex persistent pain is, and also shows us that sometimes scans or x-rays don't provide much valuable information.

One of the reasons that scans and x-rays may not paint the full picture about persistent pain is due to the fact that pain changes the way internal pain messages are sent to the brain, and a scan or x-ray cannot show these changes.

The latest research has shown us that when a person has persistent pain, there are changes in how their internal pain messaging system works. These changes affect two things:

1. How pain messages are carried around the body.

2. How the brain makes sense of the messages.

The Science of Pain

I am going to explain pain in more detail now. I have highlighted the key messages, as some of the information is complex.

The first thing that we need to know is that all pain is produced by the brain, no matter where or how it is felt.

> **There is no pain without the brain.**

Research shows that when pain persists, it is less likely to be related to ongoing injury in the tissues. Instead, 'the pathways that modulate pain (the nervous system) have become more sensitised'.

What Does this Mean?

Our nervous system is made up of:

- Our brain

- Our spinal cord (the central nervous system)

- Our nerves (the peripheral nervous system)

The body contains millions of nerves, many of which are too small to be seen on scans. The nerves have special receptors that detect changes in the body, like movement, pressure and temperature. These messages are turned into electrical impulses that are relayed to the spinal cord and the brain. The brain then has to make sense of these signals and decide if we need to respond and what that response needs to be.

Messages are constantly sent up and down these channels; the nervous system is constantly keeping up to date with the current condition of our body and what is going on in our environment.

It is a bit like a newsroom in a major TV channel when there is a constant flow of breaking news, and the news bulletins are changed and updated as that news comes in.

> ## Not all messages reach the brain.

The spinal cord can filter some of the messages and decide which ones are important enough to be relayed to the brain. Think of it like a secretary fielding phone calls; he or she decides which calls are important enough to be put through to the boss.

A Closer Look at the Brain

As we have learned, the brain receives nerve impulses from all around the body, such as pressure and chemical changes in different areas of our body. The brain weighs up this information with other important factors, like what we can see and hear, what our experiences have been, and what we know about our pain if such a signal comes in. It sorts through all of this information to decide whether or not to create a pain signal.

Why Does the Brain Do This?

The brain does all of this because its primary job is to keep us safe.

> ## Safety is of utmost importance to the brain.

Because ensuring your safety is the most important role of the brain, it is always on the lookout for something that represents a threat to you. It is like an overzealous risk assessor, or an overprotective parent, always on high alert for threat. When our brain has identified some sort of threat, it will assess the hazard and then base its response on how threatening it deems the situation to be.

If the signals are sufficient for the brain to consider them a threat, it will send a message of pain back down the nerve fibres to alert us to the fact that something has happened. This pain will continue until this 'threat' has subsided.

Why Does Pain Persist?

This is the million-dollar question – if the injury threat has gone, why has the pain not gone away? When we first injure ourselves, the pain mechanisms are temporarily turned up in that area for a short time to keep us safe and allow us time to heal. That is what happened the time I fell off the bike as a child. The pain caused me to return home and seek the care and attention of my mother. In that way, I was kept safe, and my arm had time to heal in the safety of my home.

However, persistent pain is different. Contrary to our expectations, and contrary to what many people who experience persistent pain throughout their lives assume – persistent pain does not mean that we are still injured or that we have done more damage.

A large body of research studies has shown that:

> **When you are in a persistent state of pain, your nervous system has become sensitised, meaning that you may experience pain even if there is no injury or damage to your tissues.**

Our nervous system can easily change and adapt. It will change in response to what we do, and in response to the world around us.

> **Crucially, this includes how we feel emotionally and what we know and understand about our pain.**

For example, if we have had an injury during a movement, over time, our brain can make links between that movement, the normal sensations in our body, and our memory of pain. So even though the tissues have healed, the brain (in an attempt to keep us safe) activates a pattern of nerve connections when it detects the same movement sensations in the body. If a movement is painful for long enough, these nerve connections are strengthened. The pattern of nerve connections can become sensitised and can often become sensitised enough that even *thinking* of the movement can be enough to trigger the pain response. Based on this information, we can now understand why things that normally weren't painful can start to become painful.

It may be helpful to liken this sensitised nervous system to a faulty car alarm. The car alarm should switch off and remain off unless someone is breaking into the car. A gust of wind shouldn't set the car alarm off. With persistent pain, our 'car alarm' is faulty; pain (and remember that this is 'real pain') continues to be experienced even after the injuries have healed.

This sensitisation was highlighted to me during a pain management group that I was running with a physiotherapy colleague. She was writing on a flipchart when she dropped her marker. As she bent to lift her marker, a man sitting beside her winced in pain! He hadn't moved from his chair but watching my colleague bend to lift a small object off the floor was enough for him to experience pain.

The research into persistent pain can help us explain how a person can feel pain in their left foot when they have had their left leg amputated from the knee down. Historically, we might have thought that such a person was 'imagining' the pain. We now know that they are not imagining their pain. Medical science has taught us that this problem is called 'phantom limb pain', and it is real pain. We know that there are areas in the brain which have 'memory maps' for pain. They can continue to signal pain even when there is no message coming from the original area of injury.

Thoughts and Feelings

As we have learned, body tissue does not provide the only source of information that the brain processes. Thoughts and feelings create nerve impulses too, and they make pain increase or decrease. We know that stress, and being on 'high alert' (for example, feeling anxious or worried), makes persistent pain worse. I have dedicated an entire chapter of this book (Chapter 7) to managing anxiety and stress for this reason.

Turning Down the Pain Volume

Even though research on persistent pain is constantly being carried out all over the world, we still don't know how to 'turn off' persistent pain. However, we have learned a lot of useful information about pain. While we do not have the 'off switch' for persistent pain, we do know a lot about the 'volume dial', or how to turn the volume of your pain up and down.

What is this Pain 'Volume Dial'?

Years ago, my brother had a massive red ghetto blaster radio. The radio was quite a simple device; it just had an on/off switch and a volume dial. At times, my brother turned the radio up so loud the radio shook. Now I want you to imagine that your pain is this radio. Perhaps your pain has been so intense and loud that it has vibrated and driven you to distraction. Unfortunately, as I have said several times, medical science hasn't shown us how we can turn this radio off, or cure, or turn off your pain completely. But we do know a lot about how to amplify the pain messages or how to turn the volume up on your pain. Thankfully, we also know quite a bit about dampening down the pain messages, thereby turning down the volume on your pain.

Really good illustrations of how the volume can be turned down on your pain are highlighted in the stories below.

A physiotherapy colleague of mine was doing some cross-country running in a local forest. He was running alone but had his new dog with him. He tripped on a branch and fell badly. Immediately, he felt pain in his ankle and knew he had injured himself, but fortunately, the pain was not too bad. He was far away from his car; his mobile phone had no signal, and his dog had run away. He was immediately consumed with thoughts of finding his dog and returning to his car. He managed to walk slowly back to his car and thankfully he found his dog on the way. As he approached his car, his pain went through the roof! It turned out that he had fractured his ankle and he needed surgery to fix it. Why did he not feel intense pain at the time of the accident? His brain had turned the volume down on his pain because his priority was getting back to the safety of his car and finding his dog. When his brain was sure he was safe (he could see his car), it turned up the volume of his pain as his survival was no longer a priority.

Another colleague told me a story that illustrates just how powerful our brain is in turning down the volume of our pain.

My colleague's sister-in-law was at a fancy, black-tie work event. She was strutting her stuff on the dance floor when she slipped and fell. People gathered around to assist her. Very quickly, she realised that she had lost a front tooth and rushed to the toilet. She was distraught! A colleague's wife, who happened to be a dentist, assisted her and ultimately managed to save her tooth. When the dental drama was settling down, her friend told her that she would call an ambulance. She couldn't understand why an ambulance was needed – didn't dentists deal with teeth? It was only then that she realised that she had broken both of her wrists in the fall. She had not been aware of any pain in her wrist. What had happened? Her brain had carried out its assessment, prioritised her tooth, and turned down the volume on her wrist pain.

The role that the brain plays in the pain experience can also explain how the rugby player, Joe Westerman, could continue to play an important rugby game despite sustaining a dislocated knee in the match.

In June 2019, Joe Westerman was playing for Hull FC in the British Super League (Rugby League). Playing against Hull Kingston Rovers, Westerman's knee was dislocated when his studs caught in the ground as he was tackled After carrying out 'an assessment' – his brain decided that the rugby match was more important than the pain in his knee, and as a result, the volume was turned down on his knee pain and Westerman smacked his dislocated knee back into place allowing him to play on despite his injury!

What all of these stories demonstrate is the fact that the brain seems able to turn down the volume of pain signals when it is distracted, or if it decides that other issues are more important.

Turning Up and Down the Pain Volume Dial

Scientists can be heard saying that 'our nervous system is plastic', by which they mean that it can adapt and change. This 'neuroplasticity' is illustrated when a person is recovering from a stroke. After a stroke, brain cells can regenerate, re-establish, and rearrange neural connections in response to the damage caused by the stroke. This is what happens when people who have suffered a stroke recover quite well, even after they initially lose the ability to move certain body parts or speak. The nervous system can adapt and change.

With regard to persistent pain, it has been shown that the more you understand your pain, and practise the skills that help in its management, the more your nervous system can adapt and change – in a good way. Now that we know that pain signals are released by our bodies to respond to what it believes to be a 'threat', reassuring our brains that the level of threat is minimal should help to manage the pain.

There are several other ways in which we can turn down the pain volume

- **Very gradual increases in activity and exercise levels** can turn the volume down on your pain. When you exercise, your body releases chemicals called endorphins. These endorphins trigger a positive feeling in the body, similar to morphine. The endorphins also interact with the receptors in your brain and reduce your perception of pain. If we can release more of the chemicals that feel good, we are giving our brain information that there is less threat. This reduction in threat can turn down the volume of your pain. I fully appreciate that when you live with persistent pain, it is not easy to become more active or increase your exercise level, so I have dedicated another chapter (Chapter 4) of this book to this.

- **Understanding and education about pain** are very helpful to turn the volume down on your pain.

- A large body of research evidence has shown that **mindfulness meditation** can turn the volume down (I have written more about that in Chapter 6).

- **The appropriate pacing of activity** can turn down the volume (and Chapter 5 is all about that).

- **Relaxation** can 'wind down' the nervous system and dampen pain messages.

- **Engaging in hobbies** can distract and turn the volume down.

- **Socialising and having fun** with family and friends can dampen down pain messages.

On the other hand, there are also things that can turn the volume up on your pain:

- **Stress** can turn the volume up on your pain.

- **Anxiety about your pain** can make your pain worse.

- **Anxiety about life in general** (for example, how you are going to pay your mortgage), can turn up the volume on your pain.

- **Low mood and depression** have been shown to turn the volume up.

- **Lack of sleep** makes pain worse.

- **Feeling angry and frustrated** can amplify pain messages.

- This is just a flavour of some of the things we have learned about pain management in recent years. These topics will be explored in more detail throughout this book.

Things to Remember

- Persistent pain is different from acute pain.
- Persistent pain is real pain.

- When you live with persistent pain, it does not mean that you have harmed or injured yourself further. The persistent nature of your pain is due to a more sensitive alarm system.

- Scans and x-rays may not help you or your doctor to understand why you have persistent pain.

Finally, the most important thing to remember, and the reason I felt compelled to write this book, is:

There are many things that you <u>can do</u> to turn the volume down on your pain and improve your life.

CHAPTER 2: FIND YOUR WHY

> *When we are no longer able to change our situation,*
> *we are challenged to change ourselves.*
> **Viktor Frankl**

When we think about pain management, we need to think about change. Unfortunately, change is necessary to improve your life. I use the word 'unfortunately' because – as humans – we find a change of any kind challenging... even if that is 'good' change.

I have had many periods of change in my life, and I have to say that I have often found those periods of change difficult, be it starting a new job or adjusting to having a new baby, even though that baby was much longed for.

I can think of a very simple example to illustrate this. Both my husband and I have a car. My husband's car is nicer than mine, more expensive – just a better car. I prefer to drive my car, though, and if the two cars are sitting on our driveway, I will always jump into my car. Why is that? I am drawn to my car because I am *familiar* with it. It may not be the nicer car to drive, but I know without thinking how to use all the controls, where the indicators are, and the button for the hazard lights is. When I am driving my husband's car, I have to think about where the volume dial is, where the button to heat the rear window is, and more. This feels too much like hard work, so I avoid even the simple changes that come with driving his car.

We know that change is challenging, and we also know that change is inevitable when you live with persistent pain. You have probably already had to make changes to your life. To move forward with your life, you are going to have to continue to make and adjust to changes.

> **Making positive changes to your mindset, beliefs, and behaviour can help you to better manage your pain.**

For the remainder of this chapter, I am not going to focus on talking about your pain. I think we need to set your pain aside for a moment and instead spend some time thinking about what is important to you, and the values that give meaning to your life.

Why do You Want Your Life to be Different?

Pain management often involves making changes to how you think, how you do things, and how you live your life. I am going to help you consider *why* you want your life to be different, and *why* you want to manage your pain better. I want to help you make changes to your mindset, beliefs, and behaviour, and to do that, it is necessary to first spend some time reflecting on what is important to you. These changes are a vital first step in the complete journey of managing pain.

So, why do you want to make changes to your life? Why bother doing things differently when your life is already hard enough? This chapter will focus on exploring your 'why'.

When we ponder the things that give us meaning in life, we can reflect on the life of Viktor Frankl. Viktor Frankl was an Austrian neurologist and psychiatrist who was also Jewish. In 1942, Frankl, his wife, and his parents were deported to a Nazi ghetto. In 1944, following his father's death in the ghetto, Frankl, his wife, mother and brother were moved to the Auschwitz concentration camp. Frankl's mother, brother, and wife were all murdered by the Nazis; he and his sister were the only members of his immediate family to survive the war.

When Frankl was in the concentration camp, he became interested in how people managed to live through and survive the most appalling suffering. While some people appeared to lose the will to live, others managed to cope and ultimately survive. He observed that the people who survived the camp had a sense of meaning in their lives, and this meaning helped them to survive in the most horrific circumstances and continue to live, despite their physical and emotional pain.

When the war was over, Frankl went on to write a book about his experiences, observations and philosophy entitled "Man's Search for Meaning" and it is a book that is worth reading.

You, too, are living with physical and emotional pain. While you are not living in a concentration camp, you are suffering on a daily basis. To find a way forward with your life, it is necessary to first search for the meaning in your life, the values you hold dear, your 'why'.

Studies have clearly shown that meaning in life is vitally important to well-being. Just like Frankl found in the concentration camps of Europe, studies have shown that people who have a sense of meaning and purpose – people who are living out their 'why' – cope better with the difficulties that they face in life.

What Gives Meaning to Your Life?

Life is busy. We rarely find the time to sit down and reflect on what gives our life meaning, but I think it would be beneficial for you to do so at the end of this chapter. I suggest that you read through the rest of the chapter and then set aside time to complete the written exercise below. This exercise is such a core part of your journey forward that *I urge you not to skip over it*. Give yourself the time you deserve to reflect on who you are, what drives you, what is important to you.

Please bear in mind that your values, and the things that give meaning to your life, are ***personal qualities***. Your values are individual to you. They may be different from mine; that does not mean that your values are better than mine or that mine are better than yours. They are just different. Your values define what is most important to you as an individual, and they guide the choices that you make in your life.

It is worth remembering that when you are living a meaningful, value-driven life, you are expressing your personal qualities in your daily behaviour. One of your personal values may be to contribute to the world, to help, assist or make a positive difference to yourself or others. You could live out this value in a very big way. If you found a cure for cancer, you would definitely make a positive difference to others. However, you can live out this value of contributing in more subtle ways too. You can live this value by doing small things, every day, that make a positive difference to yourself or others. This could be as simple as making a cup of tea for your partner, or letting a car out of a junction when you are in a queue of traffic.

It is not always easy to follow our values down a meaningful path, and because we are all human, we all face many doubts and struggles along the way. When I reflect on my values, I know that it has not always been a walk in the park to follow my meaningful path.

One of my values is always to continue learning and to be of service to others in the work that I do. Many years ago, in a move towards that value, I decided that I wanted to train to be a clinical psychologist. As part of my training, I was offered a place on a doctorate course. For three years, I had to get up very early in the morning, often when it was pitch dark, and drive for miles to the university where I was studying. Often, as I drove down dark, frosty, country roads, I wondered if I had made the right decision – was it worth the effort, the stress, the cost, all the hard work? My values got me through that difficult period. When I faltered and struggled, my mind was led back to my reason for the long hours and hard work, and this value, this meaning, got me through.

> **At this point, it is important to ask yourself: what values or personal qualities do I want most to express in my daily behaviour?**

Clarify Your Values

To help clarify your values, I would like you to get a notebook and pen, and go to a quiet place where you will not be interrupted. I would like you to reflect on these questions. Note down your answers. Don't worry if nothing comes to mind at first; take all the time and space that you need.

1. What do you stand for in life?

2. What do you want to do with your short time on this planet?

3. What and who matters to you in the big picture?

4. Who do you look up to? Who inspires you?

5. What personal strengths or qualities do they have that you admire?

6. What do you like to do for fun?

7. Is there anything in your life, right now, that gives you a sense of meaning and purpose, that makes you think that you are using your time in the world in a way that matters?

8. Imagine three of your closest family/friends were making speeches about you at your wedding or birthday party. Imagine them saying what you would most want to hear.

9. Who do you want to be in the world? What sort of a partner, parent, friend, colleague, etc., do you want to be?

When you have given some thought to the questions above, please complete the following exercise. And when you are carrying out the exercise, remember that we sometimes feel under pressure to resonate with a particular value because of the culture we live in, or because of our experiences in our family of origin, or some other aspect of our personal history. However, it is important to remember that this exercise is about *you* and your personal qualities. There are no 'right' or 'wrong' values; this exercise is about tuning in to what is truly important to you.

Part 1: Consider the values below. If the value listed is very important to you, *place two ticks beside it*. If the value is somewhat important to you, *place one tick beside* it. If the value is of little importance to you, *leave it blank*. I have left space at the bottom of the table for you to insert other values that are not listed here, but which are important to you.

Part 2: When you have completed the first part of the exercise, narrow down your choices to the five values that carry the most personal meaning. This can sometimes be a tricky exercise; you may find it hard to narrow things down to just five values. Don't spend too much time analysing matters, it is best just to go with your initial response. Remember, there are no right or wrong answers. Place a star beside these five values as they represent the guiding compass shining a light on what is most important in your life.

Value		Value	
Freedom		Open-mindedness	
Knowledge		Dependability	
Love		Health	
Friendship		Independence	
Justice		Authenticity	
Family		Learning	
Prosperity		Order	
Supportiveness		Patience	
Excitement		Flexibility	

Creativity		Loyalty	
Courage		Sexuality	
Power		Beauty	
Conformity		Achievement	
Control		Growth	
Honesty		Variety	
Harmony		Recognition	
Respect		Competence	
Spirituality		Persistence	
Adventure		Wisdom	
Humour		Integrity	
Productivity		Success	
Obedience		Generosity	
Responsibility		Peace	
Stability		Empathy	

Compassion		Flexibility	
Acceptance		Caring	
Kindness		Calmness	
Gratitude		Self-care	
Equality		Intimacy	
Fun		Determination	

Sometimes, people carry out this exercise with their family. You may gain some further insights doing this, so it is something worth considering but only if you feel comfortable doing this.

Over the years, I have carried out this exercise many times with a large number of people. Some people find it distressing to complete as they realise how far they have moved away from their values. For example, someone recently became tearful, stating that when they were carrying out the exercise, they realised how important it was to them to have fun in their lives. They were upset because they realised that – due to their pain and low mood – they had become more and more withdrawn, rarely engaging in anything that they found fun or enjoyable.

If this exercise has been distressing for you, it is important to remember that you should not use it as a reason to be self-critical and beat yourself up. In my experience, people who live with persistent pain are experts at self-criticism, and I will talk about this later in this book. Instead, re-frame the exercise as the beginning of your journey back to a more meaningful life.

During the remainder of this book, I will talk about values again a number of times, so don't worry if you still feel a bit confused about the concept. I will encourage you to consider making small changes in your daily life that move you towards your values and a more meaningful life; a life that *removes pain* from the driving seat, and *puts you* back in the driving seat of your life.

Things to Remember

- When you live with pain you have to change aspects of your life.

- Change is challenging.

- Reflecting on your values, the things that give meaning to your life is an important step in your pain management journey.

- Clarifying your values will help you make changes that lead you towards living a happier, more fulfilled life.

CHAPTER 3: BECOME AWARE OF YOUR INNER VOICE AND GET TO KNOW YOUR PASSENGERS

> *It is not what we say out loud that really determines our life. It is the whispers in our mind that are more powerful.*
>
> **Robert Kiyosaki**

I talk to myself. I know that you do too. I know that, because it is something that *we all do*. We all have an internal dialogue that is ongoing throughout the day. Are you aware that you talk to yourself?

> **I would like you to begin to tune into your self-talk, just notice what you are saying to yourself.**

Your mind is always chattering away, and some of your mind's chatter may be helpful. You could hear things like "You should take your umbrella with you, today, because it looks like it is going to rain," or "You can make a nice chicken stew with those ingredients," or "You can make some positive changes to your life."

However, some of the things that you hear in your mind may not be so helpful and may steer you towards decisions that lead to your world becoming smaller and smaller. They may even ultimately result in you living a 'half-life'.

It is my experience that many people have a very critical voice that dominates their chatter. This also applies to people who do not live with pain but, in my experience, it is particularly evident in people who live with persistent pain. When they tune in to what is happening in their mind, people have told me that they have heard things like "You should be able to control this pain," or "You are pathetic, you can't even work and provide for your family," or "Who would want to be in a relationship with someone like you? You are just a burden to your wife?"

Typical negative inner voices may say things like: "If you can't finish the dusting, there is no point in even starting it," or "There is no point in going for a 15-minute walk, 15 minutes walking is not going to be of any benefit," or "If you go to that party, you will have to leave early and you will ruin it for everyone else."

I could go on and on with examples of things that people have told me over the years.

Where does this 'other self' come from? As I said at the beginning of this chapter, everyone has an inner voice; you just may have never noticed it before. Essentially, this inner voice is there to protect you and keep you safe.

> **The problem is, your inner voice does not care if you are happy or living a fulfilled, meaningful life. As long as you are kept alive, and safe, its job is done.**

Many things can influence what this inner voice says, what chatter or talk your mind comes out with. If you grew up with a very critical parent or caregiver, your inner voice may be particularly critical. If you were bullied at school, your inner voice may have a lot to say – and much of it may not be very nice. If you have had other difficult childhood experiences, or if you have been abused or neglected, your inner voice can say things that are particularly unkind and unhelpful. However, even if you have not had any major adverse experiences in your life, you can still develop an inner voice that can be harsh, critical, and lacking in compassion.

> **When you live with pain, and you are making changes to your life, it is helpful to get to know and work with your inner voice.**

The first task in working with this inner voice is to begin to recognise that your mind is chattering; you need to tune in and hear your inner voice. We all can take a step back and listen to the chatter of our minds – the stories that our minds tell us. We can all work on developing our 'observer self', that part of ourselves that can listen to the chatter. But we must listen objectively without allowing our chatter to dictate our behaviour.

Imagine this scenario. You want to buy a new car, and you are car shopping with a couple of friends. Your friends and the car salesperson are giving you their opinions on what car would best suit your needs; on which car looks best, and which car has the best fuel efficiency. You can listen to their opinions, but ultimately you are the one that will be paying for the car and driving the car. Therefore, the final decision about what car to buy should be yours. You will be happiest with your new car if you have listened to the opinions of others but if *you*, and nobody else, has made the final decision about which car to buy.

When we think about how our mind works, we know that our mind is always generating ongoing chatter about what is best for us, and what actions we should take. Just like the person buying the car in the scenario above, we can choose to listen to the chatter of our inner voice, but we can decide what we want to do, how we want to behave, and what action we want to take.

Before you started reading this book, you may have been aware that you had this inner voice, chattering away all the time, or this may be the first time you have become aware of it. Either way, I would ask you to tune into it. This can seem challenging. But we can develop the capacity to become an observer of our thoughts and emotions, and this can help us move forward in our lives. Furthermore, the practice of mindfulness meditation can help us work with our inner voice. Chapter 6 of this book is dedicated to looking at mindfulness in more depth.

As mentioned, when you begin to tune into your inner voice, you will begin to notice that some of the things that your inner voice says are helpful while some things that we hear are unhelpful. But, how do we work out which is which? To help you with this, I want to direct you to your values.

If you listen to your inner voice, does it move you towards your values or away from your values? For example, let us say one of your values is to regularly connect with friends and to make some new friends. One of your friends may have invited you to their house for something (maybe for a meal) with some other people you do not know. Your inner voice may say things like, "There is no point in you going there; you will have nothing to contribute when everyone is chatting. Your life is too boring to offer anything."

When your inner voice is talking like this, the temptation is to cancel the evening, to make some excuse to get out of it. However, you have to remember that this is just an inner voice – *you can choose* to listen and take on board the advice of your mind, or you can choose to listen but ignore your mind's advice.

Your mind's chatter is essentially just a thought, and we can treat it as such; we can refuse to allow our thoughts to dictate our life. We can take ownership of our lives.

Remember, your inner voice is ultimately trying to keep you safe; in this case, protecting you from the anxiety of stepping outside your comfort zone and meeting unfamiliar people. It does not care if you are living out your values, connecting with friends, making new friends. It just wants you to stay at home where you are safe; it wants you to remain in your comfort zone.

Consider another example. You have joined a yoga class. You have never been to a yoga class before, but your friend who also lives with persistent pain has suggested it is something that might be good for you. On the morning of the class, your inner voice might be saying things like, "You are going to make a fool of yourself if you go there. You are not going to be able to do any of the poses. People will be looking at you; they will be thinking, 'What is someone like her doing here?'" If you listened to that inner voice, would you go to the yoga class? No way, of course not! But what would happen if you could tune into that inner voice; hear what it is saying, but not do as it suggests? This would mean that you make your own decision based on what you know, or suspect, will expand your life and make your life better. What if you could thank your voice for trying to protect you but decide to do something different?

This decision to observe the mind and then behave in a way that is in accordance with our values is not easy. Why? We have often spent so long listening to our inner chatter and allowing it to dictate our behaviour that we can find it hard not to believe what it says – we take it as Gospel. It is like we are hard-wired to believe everything that our mind tells us.

Throughout your lifetime, you have had millions of different experiences. As humans, we cannot remember them all. If I were to ask you to tell me about the day after your twelfth birthday, you are unlikely to be able to provide me with much detail unless something very significant happened. We cannot recall every detail because our memories do not have unlimited storage capacity.

Instead, our brains tend to selectively remember what confirms our beliefs about the world and ourselves, and they ignore the rest of our experiences. For example, you might believe that you are not good at sports. You will remember the evidence that supports that belief, and you will tend to ignore the evidence that does not support it.

A Closer Look at How the Mind Works

Imagine you are a movie editor. Your job is to watch hours of footage and to decide what to leave in the movie, what makes sense, what adds to the story. As the editor, you will leave out a lot of footage; you will leave out the scenes that don't fit in with the story.

Just like the editor of a movie, our minds edit the stories of our lives. They decide what 'scenes' to include, what makes sense to the 'storyline', and what to cut out. Our minds try to make a coherent story.

If your story is "I am useless, I cannot do anything since I developed this pain," it is possible that you will become 'fused' with this refrain and really take it on board. If this happens, you are likely to feel low and depressed, and you might shy away from trying to do things that might improve your situation. This can result in your life feeling increasingly 'smaller'.

We know that the stories our inner voice produces can be very toxic, and when people believe these toxic stories, a self-fulfilling prophecy can develop. Because the person holds on tightly to their toxic 'self-stories', they end up not trying to do something that might improve their life – perhaps not trying to become more active – "because there is no point, it wouldn't help anyway."

I want you to spend a minute imagining what the world would be like if our thoughts controlled our behaviour. It would be pretty chaotic, I fear.

We Know that Our Thoughts Do Not Control Our Behaviour

Have you ever had a thought like, "I cannot stand one more day of this pain"? If you are reading this book, you did go on to stand one more day of this pain. Even though your mind told you that you could not do it, you managed to get through and live many more days. It may not have been very pleasant, but you did it.

It is important to remember that our thoughts and stories do not control us; they do not force us to do things. Thoughts and emotions may look big and threatening at times, and it may feel as if they can control our lives, but they do not have the power to do that. Remember:

> **You are in control. You are in the driving seat of your life.**

Psychologists often use metaphors to help explain complex psychological concepts. The *passengers on a bus* metaphor is used in a therapeutic approach called Acceptance and Commitment Therapy or ACT for short. This metaphor is helpful to consider here.

I want you to imagine a bus with a lot of different passengers on it. You are driving the bus, and while some of the passengers are quiet, many of the passengers have something to say. Some of the passengers may shout at you and tell you that you are a bad driver. Another passenger may aggressively tell you to slow down as you are driving too fast; another one may tell you not to go that route as it is too dangerous. Yet another passenger may tell you that it is not worth listening to all the shouting and advise you to pull the bus over and to stop driving.

All the time, you – as the driver – can decide to listen and take on board the advice of some of the passengers, to listen to all of the passengers, or to listen to none of them. You are the driver; you decide the route, the speed of the bus, and when you want to stop and start the bus.

You may be tempted to stop the bus and try to throw all these vocal passengers off. However, there is likely to be a struggle with that; they are going to resist your efforts to shove them off the bus. Perhaps it would be better to hear them talking and shouting, but to just keep driving towards your destination. You are in control of the bus, and you decide whether you want to listen and take on the advice of the passengers.

When we consider this metaphor, now imagine that you are the driver, your mind is the bus, and the various passengers are the different stories that your mind conjures up. These stories come with a variety of emotions and urges.

At different times in your life, different passengers will be on board your bus. A significant event in your life – like the development of persistent pain – can bring new passengers, or make those passengers that were always on the bus more vocal and noisier.

It is tempting to think that we should strive only to have nice, polite, well-mannered passengers on our bus; the kind of passengers that tell you that you are a brilliant driver, that you always get things right, that you do the most wonderful job! Unfortunately, life is not like that, and none of us has a bus that is always full of those kinds of passengers.

As I write this book, there are several passengers on my bus, some pleasant, some not so pleasant. The pleasant passengers are telling me that writing this book is worthwhile; it will help some readers who are struggling to manage their pain. However, there are also some more unpleasant characters on my bus. Every so often, one shouts from the back of the bus things like, "Why are you bothering to do this? No one will want to read it." When this passenger shouts, I feel anxious and doubtful. However, I remember that I am driving my bus, I am deciding the direction I want my bus to travel, I am responsible for moving towards my values. I hear what the passenger has to say about this book, I notice that I feel anxious and doubtful, but I continue to drive my bus in the direction I choose.

It is not easy to continue driving towards our destination and our values. When the passengers are loud and threatening, our natural inclination as humans is to avoid the noise, to avoid the hard work of continuing to drive with the background noise of these loud and obnoxious passengers.

Techniques for Managing Passengers

It can be helpful to name your passengers. This can be a bit of fun, but it can also assist you with identifying who is 'talking' in your mind.

Let's imagine the case of a person named Anne, who developed persistent pain after an injury and eventually had to give up her job because of her pain. Over time, she became depressed and was struggling with anxiety. She described her pain as having taken over her life.

Anne has a very vocal passenger on her bus. This passenger has been on her bus for as long as Anne can remember; over the years, it has been more or less vocal depending on what was going on in her life.

During our conversations, Anne became aware that the passenger mentioned above was constantly putting her down, telling her that she could not do anything right. I asked her to consider naming this very critical passenger, and she decided on calling him (she thought that he was male) "Nasty Nick". Over time, she became more aware of when Nasty Nick was talking. We agreed that Nasty Nick was not all bad. He just wanted to protect her; he wanted her to remain in her comfort zone. He wanted her to remain at home, doing as little as possible in her life. This would mean she was safe.

The problem with letting Nasty Nick direct her life was that Anne rarely left the house anymore; she didn't do many of the things that she used to enjoy and her social life had dwindled.

Eventually, Anne felt well enough to look for work and she secured a new job in an employment area where she had not previously worked, but which had always interested her. In the days before she started her job, Nasty Nick was very active. He was constantly on the bus, shouting at her to reject her job offer, telling her that she would be no good at it, that it was unlike any of her previous jobs, and advising her that she would probably hate it. Nasty Nick wanted her to stay at home where she was safe. The problem was Anne did not want this; she wanted to reclaim her life, to start working again.

Even though it was very difficult, Anne managed to continue driving her bus in the direction she wanted, despite Nasty Nick's catastrophic warnings. She started her new job and found that she loved it and had a talent for this new type of work. Anne recognised that she could hear Nasty Nick, but she chose to ignore his advice. Was she anxious about starting her new job? Yes, of course, she was. Did she have doubts about whether she could do it? Yes, of course, she did. Did she sleep well the week before she was due to start it? No, she was too anxious to sleep well. Nevertheless, Anne succeeded in starting her job and moving towards her values because she recognised that Nasty Nick was on the bus, and that he was telling *the same old stories* he always told. But she did not let his voice stop her from doing what she wanted.

It can be useful to do the following exercise to get to know your mind a little more. You could try to do this over the next few days, and you could jot down some notes about the insights you have gained from doing the exercise in your notebook or journal.

- Begin to listen to the chatter in your mind and tune into your inner voice.

- Consider naming the voice; you can give it a male or female name, or if you prefer, you can give it a made-up name. Try to pick a name that resonates with you in some way and which 'fits' the voice.

- Become aware of what the inner voice is saying and appreciate that it is just 'a voice' and that you don't have to be directed by it.

- When you have become aware of your inner voice, decide what will happen if you listen to its directions. Will its directions move you towards – or further away from – the life that you want?

- Finally, become the 'driver of your bus' and decide what actions you want to take in your life.

**Know that you are the driver of your bus.
You can decide where to go
and how to get there.**

As humans, we are inclined to stay within our comfort zones, to listen to the loud, demanding passengers who insist we stay within familiar territory. As a result, we tend to resist making changes in our lives. We attempt to behave in ways that will help silence the voices in the short-term. The problem is, that does not help us over the long-term.

Let us go back to the example of going to a yoga class for the first time. If you are feeling anxious about it, and your passenger is telling you that it is a bad idea, you can give in to the demands of the passenger, park the bus and give up on trying something new. The passenger will be happy – you listened and you have done everything that he/she demanded. The anxious, fearful passenger will be quieter now, and calm will be restored in the bus for a while. But what about your destination? What about your goal of increasing your activity levels, or trying something different? What about your goal of becoming healthier? What does that mean for your pain management in the long-term? Are you paying too high a price for keeping the anxious passenger quiet?

> **We need to remember that by staying within our comfort zone, we are gaining in the short-term but we often lose in the long-term.**

When your passengers are very vocal, you may experience uncomfortable emotions, like anxiety, sadness, or anger. Nobody likes experiencing emotions like this, so we often try to push them away. Many people are fearful of experiencing strong emotions; they worry that they will fall apart or 'go mad' if they allow themselves to experience them. The difficulty is that by pushing emotions away, we often engage in behaviour that does not serve us or help us live the life that we want.

Let's look at another example. Imagine a person called Michael, who is very anxious in social situations. When he is faced with a social situation that involves meeting new people, his mind begins to tell him stories about how awful the event is going to be, how uncomfortable he will feel, how boring other people will find him, and so on. When Michael's inner voice is telling him these stories, he feels anxious. Anxiety is an uncomfortable emotion for us humans; we do not like it. Michael deals with these feelings by avoiding situations that make him feel anxious.

Michael, like many people, believes his inner voice, or 'the passengers on his bus'. Accordingly, he has developed a habit of assuming that social events are always a disaster and that people will think he is boring.

It has been important for me to work with people like Michael to help them recognise that they may experience anxiety (as uncomfortable as it is) but that they do not have to try to supress it, or allow it to dictate their social lives.

The 13th-century poet Rumi understood that our struggle to control emotions does not help us, and this is illustrated in his poem.

The Guest House

This being human is a guest house.
Every morning a new arrival.

A joy, a depression, a meanness,
some momentary awareness comes
as an unexpected visitor.

Welcome and entertain them all!
Even if they're a crowd of sorrows,
who violently sweep your house
empty of its furniture,
still, treat each guest honourably.
He may be clearing you out
for some new delight.

The dark thought, the shame, the malice,
meet them at the door laughing,
and invite them in.

Be grateful for whoever comes,
because each has been sent
as a guide from beyond.

Things to Remember

- Your mind is constantly chattering and telling stories.

- It is possible to tune in and observe what your inner voice is saying.

- Some of the things that your inner voice says are helpful and support your move towards a more meaningful life.

- Other things that your mind says are not helpful, and if you choose to listen to your inner voice *all* the time, you will move further away from the life that you want.

- Your mind likes to keep you within your comfort zone because it likes to keep you really safe. There is no need to become angry with your inner voice for this; you can thank it instead.

- Uncomfortable emotions are not dangerous; they are just part of being human. You can learn to notice them as they come and go.

- We all can make choices about whether to listen to the directions of our minds. This is our greatest freedom as humans.

CHAPTER 4: GRADUALLY BECOME MORE ACTIVE

> *Take care of your body.*
> *It is the only place you have to live.*
> **Tim Rohn**

I guess that your heart may have sunk a little when you read the title of this chapter. I also guess that you may have expected to see a chapter like this in this book.

Unless you live under a rock, you will know that physical activity is good – indeed essential – for everyone, from toddlers right through to older adults. This applies whether you have persistent pain or not. Your sinking feeling will likely be related to the fact that it is really difficult to increase activity levels when you live with persistent pain.

In this book, I use the terms physical activity and exercise interchangeably. I know that for many people, whether they live with pain or not, the word 'exercise' can be scary! For many people, exercise conjures up images of people with perfectly honed bodies, clad in lycra, doing their thing. When I use the term exercise, I mean any movement or increase in physical activity.

How Important is Exercise to You?

Before I go any further, I would like you to stop here, take out a pen and paper and write down a number, on a scale from 1 to 10. This number should reflect how important exercise, and becoming more active, is to you. 1 is not important at all, and 10 is extremely important. You can write any number from 1 to 10.

When you have done that, I want you to consider *why* you gave yourself the rating that you did. Write all the reasons that you can think of for giving yourself that rating.

The Benefits of Exercise

Let's consider the research about physical exercise and activity. We know that physical activity has very positive benefits for our physical health. Research studies have shown that regular exercise can reduce our risk of major illnesses, such as heart disease, stroke, and Type 2 Diabetes. It can also reduce the risk of some cancers by up to 50%. Regular physical exercise can lower our risk of premature death by up to 30%.

It is recommended that to stay healthy, adults should try to be active every day and aim to achieve at least 150 minutes of moderate physical activity over a week through a variety of activities. However, it is known that even small amounts of physical activity are helpful and being active for short periods of time, throughout the day, can be beneficial.

Many years ago, people living with persistent pain were advised to rest as much as possible. As more and more studies have been carried out, our understanding of persistent pain has increased. Now, people who live with persistent pain are no longer prescribed bed rest, and instead, they are encouraged to remain active.

Many guidelines that have been developed to inform practitioners how to manage persistent pain conditions have exercise at the core of the recommended treatments. For example, the 2013 Scottish Intercollegiate Guideline Network (SIGN) guidelines on the management of chronic pain recommend that, "Exercise and exercise therapies, regardless of their form, are recommended in the management of patients with chronic pain."

The National Institute for Health and Care Excellence (NICE) guidelines on the management of osteoarthritis state that exercise should be a core treatment for this pain condition irrespective of age, comorbidity, pain severity and disability. The guidelines note that exercise should include local muscle strengthening and general aerobic fitness.

We know that if you have persistent pain, exercise will improve your overall physical health and physical functioning. It is thought that exercise may help reduce the *severity* of persistent pain too. When you exercise, your body releases chemicals called endorphins. These endorphins interact with the receptors in your brain and reduce your perception of pain. This works in a similar way to the highly potent drug morphine, but without the side effects!

We know that exercise strengthens muscles. As your muscles become stronger over time, your persistent pain can feel less intense. Exercise ensures your joints keep moving well, reducing problems with stiffness; as my physiotherapy colleagues say, "motion is lotion". Exercise that improves balance and flexibility can also help reduce the risk of falls.

Research has shown us that physical activity is also very beneficial for your mental health. Studies have shown that exercise can help in the management of mild to moderate depression, as well as with anxiety and stress management. Aside from releasing endorphins, physical exercise can stimulate muscle relaxation as well as relieving tension in your body.

Many people who live with persistent pain experience sleep difficulties. I have written an entire chapter on this, but it is worth noting here that exercise can help improve sleep and that even short periods of exercise in the morning or afternoon can benefit sleep patterns. It is best to avoid strenuous physical exercise later at night as that might interfere with your sleep, but people often find that other exercise – like yoga or gentle stretching – later in the evening can help them sleep.

Many people who live with persistent pain struggle with tiredness and fatigue. It is hard to believe but becoming more active can actually help with this, and I talk about this in more detail later in this chapter.

Exercise also has a role to play in preventing and managing weight gain. Many people with persistent pain notice that they have gained weight, often due to decreased activity levels, the side effects of medication, and/or comfort eating. As well as being potentially harmful to your health, this weight gain can be a real source of distress and can have a very negative impact on self-confidence and body image.

Now that we know that regular physical activity can boost mood, improve the quality of our sleep, help with anxiety and stress, and improve energy levels, it is unsurprising that – as a psychologist – I cannot recommend the benefits of exercise highly enough! If your mental health is poor, increasing your activity levels will help you manage your mood, lack of energy, your stress and anxiety. If your mental health is good, you obviously would like to keep it that way and exercise will help you do this.

> **Without doubt, regular physical activity is one of the most powerful tools available, to help you maintain good physical and mental health.**

How Confident are You to Exercise?

I now want you to stop again, take out your pen and paper, and write a number from 1 to 10 to represent how confident you are to increase your activity levels or exercise; 1 represents very low levels of confidence while 10 represents extremely high levels of confidence.

It has been my experience that lack of confidence is where many people with persistent pain fall down. They know that exercise and increasing activity levels are important, but their confidence is in their boots; they just don't believe they can do it.

When you have written down your rating for confidence, I want you to make a list of your barriers to becoming more active, the things that stop you from exercising and increasing your activity levels. Write down as many as you can think of. I am going to address some of the most common barriers to exercise below.

Barriers to Becoming More Active

When we think about increasing activity levels, we are going to have to talk about the F word:

FEAR

As humans, we live with fear on a daily basis, yet may not even be aware of it. We turn on the news and hear about another terrorist threat, our politicians talk to us about the potential for impending economic doom – fear surrounds us.

It has been shown that fear plays a big role in persistent pain, especially in relation to activity and exercise. In my experience, one of the biggest barriers to becoming more active is anxiety or fear of making the pain worse. People live with the very real worry that increasing their activity levels or engaging in exercise is going to hurt too much, and that it is going to hurt for days after. Often, people worry that increasing activity levels or exercise may even make their pain worse indefinitely.

I think that it is entirely reasonable to experience anxiety about increasing activity levels and exercise. After all, you are suffering enough; why would you want your pain and suffering to increase?

> **Research has shown us that fear of making your pain worse through activity or exercise is very common.**

This fear of making the pain worse is so common that considerable time and effort have been spent studying it.

I would like to explore how to manage fear. When you understand fear, it becomes easier to manage. Think of something else that you are fearful of – maybe snakes, spiders, or flying. When I reflect on some of my fears, I think about my fear of jumping into the water. I was an adult before I learned to swim, and although I am a reasonably good swimmer now, I have retained my fear of jumping into the water – even the shallow end of the pool!

Consider how we deal with things that we are fearful of. Like all humans, we tend to *avoid* things that we are afraid of. Recently, I watched one of my children jump from a height into the sea on a day out. I commented to him that I would need big money, and I mean BIG money to do that. Essentially, I would avoid that activity at all cost. Luckily, my fear of jumping into water does not really affect my life; I do not get the opportunity to do it very often and my life is not affected in any negative way by avoiding it. It is similar to a fear of snakes. Thankfully we do not encounter too many snakes – at least not where I am based in the UK – so avoiding snakes has no real impact on our lives.

Avoidance of activity is different, though. Avoidance of activity can have a huge, negative impact on your life. Thinking back to the benefits of exercise that we discussed above, we know that being inactive can have significant implications for your risk of developing serious, potentially life-threatening conditions. Lack of activity can also impact negatively on your mental health. Unfortunately, it has also been established that inactivity makes persistent pain worse. The longer that you are inactive, the more likely it is that even simple, everyday tasks, like doing the housework and gardening, will become even more difficult.

When people start to become more active, they often feel pain afterwards, usually for a couple of days. This applies to people who have persistent pain and people who do not have pain. Even very fit people will experience this pain. To illustrate, let me tell you about my brother.

For several years, my brother was a professional cyclist. This meant that cycling was his main job, and as with any job, he spent many hours a day on his bike. He was super fit. One day, he decided that he was going to run on the treadmill. He was not used to running and ran for about 30 minutes. The next day his legs were really sore. Why? He had used muscles that he was not used to using. Even though he was super fit, he still experienced that pain.

I, too, have experienced that pain, which is known as 'delayed onset muscle soreness' or DOMS for short. After a two-week break from the gym, I returned to a weights class which included some squatting exercises. Even though I had been active on holiday – cycling and walking every day – I still suffered in the days after my gym class.

This means that if you have been more sedentary than normal, you are going to experience some pain when you become more active. The good news about this pain, however, is that it settles and goes away.

> **Experiencing some pain when you become more active does not mean that you have damaged yourself.**

The above statement can be hard to believe when you are stressed and worried about your pain. But it is important to remember what you have learned about pain at this point – pain is a signal of harm or damage. But, remember that this *only* applies to acute pain, not long-term persistent pain.

The muscle soreness that sometimes occurs when starting a new exercise or becoming more active subsides as your body adapts to the new activity levels. This short-term increase in pain or soreness can be minimised if you pace your activity. Please remember that a temporary increase in pain, due to a lack of pacing, does not mean that you have harmed yourself. I will talk about pacing in depth in the next chapter,

It is remarkable how quickly the human body can become 'deconditioned'. When somebody has become deconditioned, it means that multiple, potentially reversible changes have occurred in the body system due to physical inactivity and disuse. Have you ever seen an arm or leg that has just come out of plaster after a break? If you have, you will notice that it is thinner and weaker than the other limb. This happens after only a few weeks of being immobilised in plaster. If you have been living with pain for months and years, and have become gradually more inactive over that time period, you may have become deconditioned. This can partly explain why even normal day-to-day activities have become harder. The good news is that as you increase your activity levels, your muscles will become stronger!

Managing Fear and Anxiety

We need to consider the best way to deal with the anxiety that you feel about increasing your physical activity levels. I realise that your doctor, your physiotherapist, or myself could reassure you ('til the cows come home) that activity will not harm you, but there will always be a part of your brain that does not believe it. This is simply because we have all been programmed from a young age to believe that pain means harm.

Think back to what I told you about my fear of swimming. I had swimming lessons at school with the rest of my class, right through secondary school. I was the only one left at the age of 18 that could not swim. How embarrassing was that? My friends all reassured me, "You won't drown; the PE teacher and the lifeguard are here." Did I believe them? No, I did not!

I can now swim quite well, easily swimming a kilometre. What miracle occurred to allow that to happen? It was quite simple, really. I was highly motivated to overcome my fear of swimming. I wanted to learn how to participate in something that looked like it was great fun. Later in life, I wanted to be that mum that could go into the pool with her children.

As a student, I spent a summer working in America. We lived beside the sea and I started going to the beach every day to practise swimming. I swam in very shallow water. Even I knew I couldn't drown in that. Gradually, I learned to swim and became more and more confident, moving to deeper and deeper water. By the end of the summer, I had realised my dream and I could swim.

As psychologists, we use these principles all the time when we help people to overcome their fears or phobias; this method is known as 'graded exposure'.

To overcome your anxiety about movement, you need to apply the same principles. Start with very small steps (shallow water) and gradually increase your activity levels (move to deeper water) as your confidence increases. The only way that you can really appreciate that activity will not harm you is by *doing it and seeing what happens*. I do not believe that anyone could ever really 'talk' you out of that strongly-held belief that increasing activity levels will hurt and that it will continue to hurt every time you do it. So I urge you to try, very slowly and gradually, to increase your activity level and see for yourself what happens.

Over the years, I have worked with many people who have faced their fears about increasing their activity levels with great courage. I am not being condescending; it takes great courage to face your fears. All of them realised that it is safe and achievable to increase their activity levels and live a better, healthier life. Many of these people became more active by very gradually increasing the time or distance that they walked. Others started going to the pool, some to swim, others to walk in the water. Some people joined a yoga class, others started becoming more active by walking up and down their stairs a couple of times more a day.

While fear is the biggest barrier to increasing activity levels for people who live with pain, there are often other barriers to increasing activity levels, too. I have listed some other barriers below.

I Don't Know What Exercise to Do or Where to Start

It is beyond the scope of this book to advise you exactly how you can increase your activity level. The type of activity or exercise that you want to engage in is entirely up to you. You may choose to increase your walking (a step counter watch can be highly motivating). I have been known to walk around the house a few times before bed to meet my step target!

Conversely, walking may not suit you, depending on where your pain is. You may decide that swimming is for you. Others may try cycling, dancing, yoga, chair-based yoga, pilates; the list is endless.

There are certain exercises that you may decide are not for you; they don't suit you and your pain. That is fine; there are so many alternatives out there that you will always find something that suits your particular circumstances.

As I said previously, *any activity is a good activity*, providing you enjoy it and it suits you. There is no point in considering swimming if you are terrified of the water. There is little point in trying to go to a yoga class if you hate every second of it. You may have to try several different activities or exercise until you find one that suits you and that you enjoy.

There are great resources online; all you need is your phone or laptop and YouTube. Indeed, there are numerous really good YouTube exercise videos available, but be sure to try out the beginner's versions if you have been inactive for a while. Also, remember that you do not need to 'complete' a video; you may only be able to do a minute or two. A minute or two is a great start; if you keep with it, you will soon see progress!

Many people reading this book may feel that they need professional support to help them increase their activity levels. If you have become very inactive because of your pain, if your confidence to exercise is very low, or if you are very anxious about exercise increasing your pain levels, consider requesting a referral to a physiotherapist for support and advice. Physiotherapists are the experts in helping people become more active, and they can provide you with good advice on how to begin to move more. I can assure you that a physiotherapist will be delighted to hear you say that you need their help to become more active. Reach out for the available help – you will not regret it.

It can also be helpful and motivating to incorporate a social element into your activity. Walking or exercising with your partner, family member, or friend can be a great way to connect. I always find that the time flies when I am walking with a friend as I am so busy talking I do not even notice that we are walking. You may not be able to walk as far or as fast as your friend, but that is okay. You can choose to work around this by agreeing to walk for a shorter period of time, or by resting on a park bench while your friend does another lap.

If you decide to go to a class in your local gym or community centre, make sure to go a little bit earlier the first day so that you can tell the physiotherapist or instructor that you have a persistent pain problem. That way, they can keep an eye on you in the class and recommend an alternative exercise or pose if you find one of them particularly challenging. It is pretty normal for at least one person in every exercise class to have a specific difficulty, which means that part of the class has to be adapted for them. Also, remember you do not have to do every exercise in a class.

You may also have to stop and start frequently. Again, this is very common; people have to do this all the time – people who do not have persistent pain do so, too. The most important thing is that you are working on improving your activity levels, and by doing so, you are building your fitness, improving your pain management, and opening yourself up to all the health benefits of exercise.

Work Out Your Baseline

Some people reading this book may be quite active currently; perhaps walking, cycling or swimming regularly. Others will be extremely inactive. To figure out how to become more active, you need to establish your baseline first and then very gradually increase your activity levels.

Reading Chapter 14, which discusses goal setting, will help you with this. It has been my experience that people who live with pain can often set unrealistic and unachievable activity goals. They do this because they think about their 'old', pre-pain self when they are setting their goals. For example, if you regularly went to the gym before you developed your pain, you may set yourself goals that are too hard to achieve because it is difficult to accept what your new baseline is. If you set your goals too high, you will not be able to achieve your goal, or if you do achieve it, you may notice a significant (but temporary) increase in your pain that lasts several days. This can then add to your sense of hopelessness and disempowerment; when you experience these things, you are likely to give up trying.

After you have chosen a particular exercise or activity, you can use the following steps to work out what your baseline with the activity/exercise is. You can then set achievable goals from there.

Let's use the example of walking. If you can walk for 10 minutes without any significant increase in your pain, you may decide to set the goal of walking for 10 minutes – three times a week – for your first week.

You may subsequently decide to increase the time you spend walking by 1 more minute the following week, or you may decide to remain at 10 minutes until you build up your confidence or until your body adjusts to the increased activity levels. Staying at the same level for some time is still progress – all the time, you are building your fitness – but more importantly, you are building your confidence and you are learning that it is safe to move more.

I Don't Have The Energy

Many people who have persistent pain struggle with their energy levels. This can be particularly true for people who live with

Fibromyalgia, but difficulties with energy are commonly reported by people who live with all types of pain. We know a lot of the medication that is prescribed for people with persistent pain have unpleasant side effects and one of these side effects is feeling sedated and low in energy. Also, if your mood is low and you are depressed, your energy may also be reduced.

It sounds counter-intuitive, but we know that one of the best ways of improving energy levels is to become more active. However, it is best to do that gradually (as described above) as this makes it more likely that you will persist with your increased activity levels or exercise. As I mentioned earlier, our bodies very quickly become deconditioned when we are inactive. As a result, even simple tasks like taking a shower and getting dressed can be exhausting. Research has shown that this lack of energy will improve over time with gradual increases in activity levels and the associated improvements in physical fitness.

It can be helpful to *schedule* your exercise or physical activity at the time of the day when your energy is at its highest. You may decide, also, to break up your daily exercise into two or three different sessions during the day. For example, you may find that doing 10 minutes of yoga in the morning and 10 minutes in the evening suits you. Experiment with the timing and find what suits you and your body best.

Try to find ways to sneak in a bit of extra activity when you can – it all adds up. Park the car a little bit further from the door of the supermarket; take the stairs if you can manage them. Even taking one flight of stairs before using the lift for the rest of your journey is progress. Let go of the idea that exercise needs to involve a gym or a lot of sweating.

I Don't Have The Motivation

This is one of the most common reasons why people don't exercise. To address this, I think it is important to first reflect on your values; your reasons for doing things that are difficult, your reasons for making changes that take a lot of effort. Why are you bothering to read this book? Why did you buy it? I suspect that you are reading this book because you are fed up living a 'half-life'. You want a change. You want things to be different. For your life to be different – for your life to improve – you are going to have to make some changes to what you do; you are going to have to try some new things.

> **If you do what you have always done, you will get what you have always got.**

People aren't born motivated. They become motivated. They think about the reasons *why* they want to do the difficult things; they consider them to be challenging, and they start to do those difficult things. Over time, their confidence begins to grow; they continue to do the difficult things, and one day they wake up and notice the things that were once very challenging have now become a lot easier. They are motivated to continue; the motivation has followed the action.

To improve your motivation to increase your activity levels, it can be really helpful to write down your reasons for making changes to your life and read them aloud every morning and every night before bed. If you have not completed the values exercise in Chapter 2 you should think about doing so; it will help you come up with your list of reasons for changing.

Lastly, do not overthink things! Nike came up with the slogan 'Just do it' for a reason. Often, we can talk ourselves out of something; it is so easy to put off making changes, to delay going for that walk or going to that yoga class. We tell ourselves that we will do it in half an hour, or this afternoon, or next week, or next month, or next year. Now is the only time you have... so just do it!

I Don't Have The Time

Lack of time is a widespread barrier to becoming more active or starting to exercise. Again, I would ask you to reflect on your values and your list of reasons for making changes to your life. Everyone has the same 24 hours in a day and, as individuals, we decide every day how to spend that time. Often, we get into a rut of spending time on things that feel good but which ultimately do not add anything much to our lives or move us towards our values.

Binge-watching Netflix, or scrolling through Facebook and Instagram is enjoyable and, of course, there can be a place for all of that in our lives, but we need to think about the time we spend doing things that do not add *real value* to our lives.

If we decide that we want to incorporate 20 minutes of exercise, three times a week in our life, we need to decide what else has to give: do we spend 20 minutes less on our phone; do we give up time watching the news on TV?

Even the busiest of people have time to prioritise activity and exercise. I remember reading an article about Barrack Obama. When he was the US President, he *made time* to exercise regularly as well as go on a 'date night' once a week with his wife. I think if the US President can do it, we all can!

I Am Too Embarrassed to Exercise

This is a barrier to exercise that I have come across many times during my work. In conversations with friends, I have also come across this concern often. I can recall one friend tell me that she avoided going out for a walk because she was worried about what people passing by in cars would think about her. Specifically, she worried that people would think things like, "Look at the state of her, that walking is not doing her much good!" I have heard other people say that they would never use a gym because they are overweight; that they would only use a gym if they lost a stone or two first.

Many people have told me that they would love to try swimming again; they enjoyed it in the past and they felt that it was something that they could maybe try once more. However, many explained that they felt too uncomfortable being seen in public in a swimming suit or shorts. This embarrassment about their body was so great, they would not even consider going to the swimming pool.

People who experience pain are often embarrassed about how slow they walk, or the fact that they have to use a stick or a crutch. People who feel like this typically avoid exercising and even walking in public. I have worked with people who have even avoided going out to shopping centres as they did not want anybody to see them walking slowly or using a crutch or a stick.

When you let embarrassment direct your behaviour, when you let embarrassment determine whether you go out for a walk, join a gym, go to the swimming pool, or go shopping, you are closing down your life. You are moving away from a rich, full life and closer to a life in which many enjoyable activities no longer feature.

Again, I am going to ask you to consider your values; we are constantly going to go back to them because this is your roadmap to a better life, a fuller life. Are you letting your feelings of embarrassment, or fear, or worry prevent you from doing the things that you *know* will lead you towards a better life? If you are, you need to consider the price you are paying for allowing these emotions to dictate your behaviour, your choices in life.

> *Care about what other people think and you will always be their prisoner.*
> **Lao Tzu**

If you live your life in an attempt to control what other people may (or may not) think about you, you will end up living a very small life. This is true whether you live with persistent pain or not.

As humans, we are conditioned to care about what other people think about us; it is innate in us to work in 'packs', to live in groups. That is one of the reasons the human race has flourished. However, it can be detrimental to our wellbeing to become too concerned about what others think about us, especially when our concerns move us away from our values and a meaningful, full life in the way described above.

It is also helpful to consider another tendency that all people have; the tendency to be a mind reader, *the tendency to think that we know what other people are thinking.* Psychological research has shown that we all make 'cognitive errors' or, simply put, we make mistakes in how we interpret information about what is going on around us.

One of the most common errors that people make is to think that they know what other people are thinking, and often this is interpreted negatively. This is particularly true if you have been feeling anxious, low, or depressed. You could look at someone and be convinced that they are thinking that, "He is too young to have that stick," or "Look at the state of her in that swimsuit!" It is important to recognise that these are unhelpful thoughts and they may hold you back from going to the shopping centre again or going back to the swimming pool.

> **If you let negative thoughts direct your behaviour, are you going to be able to live a full life?**

Later in this book, we will talk about how to manage thoughts like the above in more detail. However, it is worth remembering that, as individuals, we mindread all the time, but only a very, very small number of people, who appear on TV and in shows in Las Vegas, are any good at it!

Things to Remember

- Physical activity is extremely important for our physical and mental wellbeing.

- When we exercise, our body releases endorphins. Endorphins are the body's natural pain killers.

- Anxiety or fear about making the pain worse is the most common barrier to increasing activity levels.

- The fear of making pain worse can be overcome by *slowly* and *gradually* increasing activity levels.

- A physiotherapist can provide expert help on increasing activity levels if required.

CHAPTER 5: BECOME A RULE BREAKER

> **Sometimes, breaking the rules is necessary. It is ok to break the rules when doing so leads you closer to the life that you want to live.**

As humans, we use rules to govern our behaviour. From a young age, you will have learned numerous rules; for example, always be polite to strangers, do not burp in public, wash your hands after you use the toilet, and do not talk with your mouth full!

These rules can be useful as they help us function in society. However, they can also be problematic if they are *always* followed rigidly, or if they are followed when they no longer serve us or add value to our lives.

The Homemaker

Let's use Michelle's experience as an example. Since she developed her pain, some of Michelle's rules had become very problematic for her – they no longer added value to her life. Michelle had a rule that her home must be clean and tidy at all times. She also had the rule that every item of laundry that was washed needed to be ironed (including things like underwear, socks, towels and bedsheets). Also, the rule was that the ironing was done on the day that the washing was done. These rules were not particularly problematic for her before she developed her pain. Even though cleaning and ironing were time-consuming, she previously managed them without any significant difficulties.

However, when Michelle developed Fibromyalgia, she was frequently exhausted and in pain. Despite her pain and her exhaustion, Michelle continued to live by her rules – the house must be clean and tidy at all times, and everything must be ironed on the day that it is washed. This became difficult for her because following these rules meant she had to spend many hours every week cleaning, tidying, and ironing.

Like most people who live with pain, Michelle experienced good days and bad days with her pain and fatigue. Some days, she was particularly sore and tired. However, even on her worst days, she lived by her rules and continued to do her cleaning, tidying, and ironing – taking as few breaks as possible. Following the rules meant that Michelle felt exhausted and sore, and she was left without enough energy to do some of the things that were really important to her – like spending time with her children. Typically, Michelle went to bed around 7 pm every evening; she felt like she could not stay up a moment longer. She was upset by this. She spent less time with her family than she would have liked, especially her children as they were only home from school for a couple of hours before she went to bed.

I spent some time discussing these rules with Michelle and reflecting on how they were serving her. She was *very resistant* to changing them; her mother had taught them to her many years ago, and she had always lived by them. There were benefits to this way of living, her house was clean and tidy, and her clothes were ironed to perfection. However, she also recognised that she paid a heavy price for following the rules so rigidly.

Michelle decided to make some changes to her rules because she recognised that she would free up time to spend with her children. By spending more quality time with her children, she was moving towards one of her most important values – *being emotionally and physically available to meet her children's needs*. In short, she decided to no longer iron small items, towels, or sheets, and to relax her rules about always keeping the house clean and tidy. These 'rule breaks' allowed her to conserve her energy for the things that were more important to her.

Now, let us consider Jim's experience.

The Gardener

One of Jim's rules was that 'you always cut the grass in the front and back lawn on the same day'. This was a longstanding rule for him, but (like Michelle in the previous example), this gentleman came to realise that this rule no longer served him. Yes, Jim could do the front and back lawn on the same day. However, he paid a hefty price for doing so when he was sore for days afterwards.

Because Jim was sore, he was irritable with the people around him and his relationships suffered as a result. Like most people, he took out his frustration and pain on the people closest to him, often his partner. This caused him to feel guilty, and this guilt further added to his distress and suffering.

By breaking his rule about mowing the lawn, Jim found that he could manage his pain better; he was able to break this physically demanding job into more manageable chunks. He decided that he would cut the front lawn one day, and cut the back lawn another day. As a result, he was not as sore and irritable, and he was moving towards an important value concerning the type of relationship he wanted with his partner.

This rule-breaking was not without a price... rule-breaking rarely is! Jim was aware of his rule about always completing a job once it was started; it was passed down to him from his father who frequently counselled him, "Don't bother starting a job unless you are prepared to finish it." Jim had internalised this rule; he adopted it as a rule for life, and he held this rule rigidly in his mind.

Like many of the rules that we live by, Jim was *not even aware* of having this rule until he took the time to sit down and reflect on his life. When he began to 'rule-break', Jim had to live with the anxiety of having done an incomplete job; starting a job one day and completing it the next day, or even a couple of days later.

As you would expect, Jim's mind had plenty to say about the matter! In his mind, he heard things like, "You are just being lazy. You can finish the lawn; just get on with it." His mind even provided weather warnings, "What are you going to do if it rains tomorrow? You are not going to get it done then!" There were also comments about what the neighbours might say, "The neighbours are going to be talking about you. They will be wondering what is wrong with you when you can't even finish the lawn."

Our mind is a very persuasive storyteller and it can be hard to cope with stories like this. We are programmed to believe what our minds tell us and to conform to their demands. However, Jim decided not to take on board the comments of his mind; he thanked his mind for its stories, but he decided to do something different, to do something that moved him towards his values. He allowed the stories in his mind to become background noise; he allowed his mind to chatter on but he chose not to pay attention to it.

Psychologists describe this type of rule-breaking behaviour as *psychological flexibility*.

> **Psychological flexibility is about becoming aware of what is important in life, and changing – or persisting – in your behaviour in the service of your chosen values.**

There have been hundreds of studies carried out on psychological flexibility, and there is really good evidence that this flexibility is associated with positive outcomes for people, whether they live with pain or not.

At this point, I would like you to take some time out and jot down in your notebook or journal some of the rules that you live with. This may seem challenging at first; just like Jim in the example above, you are probably not even aware of the rules that you live by. To make this task a little easier, it might be helpful to think about some of the rules that your parents had, as it is likely that they passed these rules onto you. If you did not grow up with your parents, think about the rules that your primary caregivers lived by.

When I reflect on my own life, I am aware that one of my parents' rules was that "Even if you don't feel well, you make every effort to go to work or school." I have no memory of my parents ever verbally passing this rule onto me, but I am aware that my parents lived by this rule and encouraged their children to live by it, too. Thankfully, I am rarely unwell, but when I am unwell, this rule comes into play. I struggle to take time off work to recover because my mind is very quick to point out that "You should be at work, even if you don't feel well."

When you are compiling your list of rules, you might notice that a lot of them have the words like **should, must** or **have to** in them.

- I **should** be able to work full-time and provide for my family.

- I **must** do all my housework on a Friday.

- I **must** do my grocery shopping all in one go.

- When I am at work, I **have** to be performing at 100% at all times.

- I am only 30 years old. I **should** be able to walk for half an hour without stopping for a rest.

- I **have** to get rid of my pain before I can live my life.

- I **have** to have a tidy and clean house at all times.

- I **should** not ask other people for help.

- I **must** be the person who everyone comes to for help in the family.

- I **should** be able to work out for an hour in the gym.

These rules often incorporate 'all or nothing thinking'. Alex's story illustrates this.

Alex was very fit and active before he developed his pain. Being physically active and maintaining a high level of fitness was a core part of his job, and he also enjoyed playing sports outside of work. He had been a champion sportsman in his younger years, and performing on the sporting field – at the highest level possible for his age – was very important to him. Alex's self-worth was very much tied to his perception of himself as a man who was at the 'top of his game' physically.

This did not cause Alex any problems until he had an injury and was unable to perform to these high standards. Despite his pain, he knew that he could be physically active and take part in some exercise classes, albeit at a lower level than he did previously. However, Alex used 'all or nothing' thinking when he considered going back to exercise, admitting that he often thought, "If I can't compete at the highest level, there is no point in doing any gym classes." His rule that he had to compete at the highest level was no longer serving him, but he struggled to modify his exercise regimen, and as a result, had become inactive and depressed.

After our discussions, Alex recognised that he was thinking in an 'all or nothing' way, and that he had been living by the rule that you had to perform at the highest level. He recognised that even though he could not perform at a high level because of his pain, he should not give up doing any physical exercise, but instead enjoy doing what he could.

Back to You

When you have compiled your list of rules, reflect on them and decide which rules continue to serve you and add meaning to your life. Also, decide which rules no longer add anything to your life; identify those rules that move you away from your values. You may notice that some of your rules have *never* really served you in life, and that this was the case even before you developed your pain.

Remember Michelle from the story above? After some time, she realised that her cleaning, tidying, and ironing rules did not really serve her, even *before* she developed her Fibromyalgia. She realised that her rules had been rigid and extreme, even when she had the energy to follow them. She could recall friends coming over to visit, and being unwilling to take time out to sit and have a coffee with them as she was on a tight schedule to complete the cleaning and ironing activities that her rules demanded. Instead of sitting with them, she stood – ironing – while she chatted to them. When she reflected on this, she realised that even before she developed her pain, her rules moved her away from her values.

When you have written your list of rules, decide what rules you want to modify or completely let go of.

Recognise that this is often not an easy process; your mind is likely to have plenty to say about it! But also recognise that you are in the driving seat of your life. You, *not your mind*, can decide what you want to do with your life and how you want to live.

The Three Ps

When we think about pain management, we often talk about the 3 Ps. The first P is for pacing, the second one is for planning, and the third one is for prioritising.

I remember being a member of a gym and on the wall, beside a painting of a man rippling with muscles, was the sign "No Pain, No Gain". The purpose of this sign was to motivate people to push past their pain threshold, to do a few more reps of their weight exercises, to do a few more sit-ups, to squeeze in a few more push-ups, despite the pain. Even if you have never set foot in a gym in your life, you will probably be familiar with the saying.

It is my experience that some people who live with persistent pain adopt a "No Pain, No Gain" attitude when they think about their pain. They convince themselves that if they could only 'push through' that everything will be ok, that they will minimise the impact that their pain has on their lives. Unfortunately, while this mantra may be useful for bodybuilders in the gym, it does not work for people who live with persistent pain.

To illustrate this, let me tell you a story about a lady who we can call Maggie.

The Mother

Maggie (like Michelle) lived with the persistent pain condition of Fibromyalgia. As is common with all persistent pain conditions, Maggie had good and bad days with her pain. While she never had a day in which she was pain-free, some days she did not feel too bad. On other days, though, her pain was debilitating.

Maggie had worked hard all her life. She had a part-time job, she was a single mother and cared for her children, and she managed her home. Maggie had to give up her part-time employment due to her pain, but she remained in her full-time role of mum and housekeeper.

On bad days, Maggie was limited in what she could do. She did the essentials, making sure that her children had clean clothes to wear and she prepared meals for them to eat. These days were hard for Maggie; she felt guilty and frustrated that she could not do more. The children asked to go to the swimming pool and she was too sore to get into the water with them. The windows needed to be cleaned and she could not do them as she was in too much pain. The kitchen cupboards were a mess but her condition prevented her from cleaning and tidying them.

Of course, Maggie had good days too. There were days when she got up in the morning and her pain wasn't too bad. On those days, Maggie decided to go for it; she had wasted enough time on her pain. On those days, Maggie did all her normal chores, but she also tackled the kitchen cupboards, the windows, and her daughter's messy bedroom. Maggie noticed that by early afternoon, she was exhausted and had become really sore again, but she adopted the "No Pain, No Gain" motto and decided to push through and finish her daughter's room. How do you think Maggie felt the next day?

Typically, the next day and for a few of the following days, Maggie felt awful. Her pain flared up, and she was back to doing the minimum needed to keep her family ticking over. Maggie continued in this 'boom-bust' cycle for a long time. She felt increasingly frustrated, hopeless, and guilty – stating that her pain and fatigue had completely taken over her life.

The difficulties experienced by Maggie are illustrated in the diagram below.

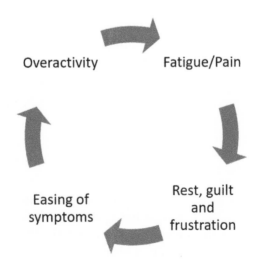

Overactivity

Fatigue/Pain

Easing of symptoms

Rest, guilt and frustration

The scenario described above is known as the boom-bust cycle, and I want you to determine if this sounds familiar to you in any way. While your situation may be very different from Maggie's situation, you may notice that you tend to tell yourself to always push through the pain. As a result, you may notice that you have days when you are quite inactive and days when you are very active.

I am going to tell you another story. This time, it is about a man called Paul.

The Provider

Like Maggie, Paul had worked all his life, starting work on a building site at the age of 16. He had loved working and did not mind the 12-hour days. When he was in his mid-40s, he developed back pain. He hoped it would resolve; he had experienced episodes of back pain in the past, but his pain always got better.

Within a few years, however, Paul was struggling. His pain had not gone away and he was no longer able to work. The loss of his job was a massive blow for Paul. He had prided himself on his work ethic and was gratified that he could provide a good home and lifestyle for his family.

He became depressed and withdrew from his friends and family, and spent most of his day watching TV. He tried to become more active but every time he made the effort, he noticed that his pain got worse. Over the years, Paul stopped trying, and – like Maggie – he felt frustrated and guilty. He was also angry that his life had turned out this way. He described his life as being like that of a 90-year-old man confined to home due to ill health.

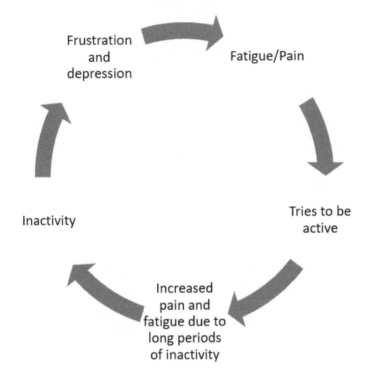

Frustration and depression → Fatigue/Pain → Tries to be active → Increased pain and fatigue due to long periods of inactivity → Inactivity → Frustration and depression

You may find that aspects of Paul's story are familiar to you. You may notice that you have become very inactive due to your pain. You may recognise the emotion of frustration and the experience of depression.

You will also notice that even though Maggie and Paul coped differently with their pain, they both experienced increased levels of pain and fatigue as well as feelings of frustration.

Fortunately, there is a pain management skill that is of great benefit to Maggie and Paul, despite their different ways of coping. It is known as *pacing*.

Pacing

Pacing can be applied to many different types of activity; it can be used with housework, self-care tasks, gardening, studying, and paid work. There is good research evidence for the benefits of pacing across a variety of pain conditions including, Fibromyalgia, neuropathic pain, and the pain associated with arthritis.

Pacing is essentially taking a break in your activity *before* you need it; before the volume in your pain is really turned up. Over time, pacing can help you become more active.

Learning to Pace, Finding your Baseline

How do you learn to pace? Essentially, pacing involves breaking down any physical activity – whether that is going for a walk, preparing a meal, decorating a room, or sitting working on a computer – into manageable chunks.

First, consider what position your body is in when you carry out the activity. For example, washing dishes involves standing, studying for an exam involves sitting, sweeping the floor involves standing in a flexed-forward position.

Next, consider how long you can be in this position before you notice that your pain increases. Although it may seem tedious, it is worth using the stopwatch or timer on your phone to work this out.

Once you have established your baseline figure, it is recommended that you then reduce this figure by 20% and start to use this new figure as a baseline for this particular type of activity or exercise.

To illustrate some of the challenges that you are likely to experience when you start to pace your activity, I want to tell you about Jack.

The Hiker

Before he developed his pain, Jack was very active. He worked in a physically demanding full-time job, often doing overtime as well. At the weekend, he enjoyed hiking, and most weekends went for a four-hour hike on a local mountain range.

When he developed his pain, Jack tried to continue working for as long as possible. However, he got to the point where he just could not continue with work, and he was forced to give up his job. Unfortunately, he could not continue hiking either, due to his pain. Over a few years, he became depressed and very inactive.

Jack realised that getting out of the house and walking or hiking was important to him and that it helped his mental health. However, Jack found it difficult to accept that he could no longer go on his four-hour hikes. He tried to cut his walking back, typically going on a shorter one-hour hike, but he found that his pain went through the roof the next day and for the days that followed. As a result, he restricted his activity levels in an attempt to get his pain under control. When his pain settled, he tried to go back out for his hour-long walk again. And so, the boom-bust cycle continued – his pain increased significantly, and he then restricted his activity until it settled.

Jack was advised to pace his walking in the hope that he could gradually increase the time and distance he could walk. Jack timed his walking over three days. The first day that he timed it, he worked out that he spent 30 minutes walking before his pain significantly increased. The second day, he walked for 35 minutes before his pain increased. The third day, he was a bit sore in the morning and after 25 minutes of walking, he noticed his pain levels starting to increase. Based on this information, by getting the average of the three figures, he worked out that he could walk for 30 minutes without his pain increasing significantly.

When he reduced the 30 minutes by 20%, his baseline of walking for 24 minutes was set. Jack was encouraged to use this baseline of 24 minutes. It was recommended to Jack that – even if he felt he could walk further – he should remain with the 24-minute baseline figure for the first week. If he felt good, he should gradually increase that figure over the coming weeks by about 10% per week.

Initially, the baseline figure of 24 minutes made Jack feel frustrated and angry. After all, he was used to much longer hikes. However, he also recognised that his boom-bust strategy was not working for him. So, Jack decided to take the advice on board, and he started to pace his walking exercise.

Jack's biggest challenge to pacing were the stories that his mind generated about it. His inner voice continually told him to push on, to walk a bit further, that it was ridiculous to stop. Jack had spent a lot of time living with the rule that there was no point in doing any exercise unless you worked up a sweat and pushed yourself. Eventually, Jack was able to ignore what his mind was saying and continued with pacing. He became a rule-breaker and broke his old "No Pain, No Gain" rule about exercise. Jack realised that this rule no longer served him; it was making his life more difficult, pushing him into this boom-bust cycle.

After several months of pacing his exercise, Jack was walking faster and for longer distances. His fitness had improved and he felt more positive and confident. Jack didn't experience as many flare-ups and – when they did occur – they didn't last as long.

You will notice that Jack worked out his baseline for walking and – importantly – that he didn't go beyond his baseline, despite what his mind told him. Instead, he slowly increased his activity levels beyond his baseline over weeks and months. It is crucial to note that if Jack had stayed at his baseline, without slowly and steadily increasing his activity levels, he would not have made any significant improvement in his fitness levels.

Increasing your Activity after you Establish your Baseline

You can move forward with your activity levels in many ways. Like Jack, you may choose to increase the time you spend doing an activity. Alternatively, if you engage in any type of weights or resistance activity, you may choose to increase the weight or resistance that you are lifting or pushing. You may choose to work on reducing the rest time between your activities. All of these approaches are fine; it is just about finding which ones work for you.

It is important to remember that your baseline for activity may be very short. I have worked with many people whose baseline was several minutes. *It doesn't matter* what your baseline is – it could be 60 seconds, it could be four hours – pacing is applicable no matter how active or inactive you are.

When carrying out activities, it is worth remembering that changing your position can also be helpful. Take dinner preparation as an example. You may find it helpful to stand for 10 minutes to cut vegetables and then move to a seated position to cut some more vegetables. Just because you have never sat at a table when cutting vegetables does not mean that this will not work for you.

Like many of the tools in this book, it can be very helpful to keep a written record of your progress. Record your baseline figures and log how you progress from there. Please remember that pacing, like all pain management strategies, is not a magic wand that will provide instant results. However, if you can be patient and compassionate towards yourself, *you will get results*.

Planning

As I noted earlier in this chapter, we often talk about the 3 Ps of pain management. The first P is for pacing, and the second one is for planning, which I will discuss now.

Planning your activities is helpful when you are living with persistent pain. Most people who have lived with pain for a while recognise that planning activity is one of the things that they have to do.

My patients consistently tell me that the necessity of planning activity is one of the most frustrating aspects of living with pain. I can understand this frustration. In your life before pain, you could, within reason, spontaneously decide to go on a day trip, go out for the evening, or do some other activity on the spur of the moment. When you live with pain, you are likely to have to be a bit more thoughtful about your level of activity. For example, if you have had a very active day and a friend texts you to ask if you want to go out for something to eat, you may have to decline their offer because you are too tired and/or sore.

The need to plan more carefully is common with other chronic health conditions. If you have diabetes, you need to carry your blood testing kit, insulin, and sugary food or drink to treat hypoglycaemia. You also need to plan your meals more than someone who does not have diabetes. As with other chronic conditions, the sooner you accept that planning makes your life easier, the easier your life will become in the long run.

Planning activity when you have persistent pain can prevent the escalation in pain that is common with boom-bust activity cycles. For example, if you have friends coming to stay for a few days, you may have to start planning for their visit well before their arrival. You may have to change a bed or prepare somewhere for them to sleep, shop for extra food, and do other activities that you do not normally do. You may also know that you are going to be more active when they are staying with you, perhaps going out for dinner or taking a day trip with them. If you leave all the preparation to the day before their arrival, you are likely to experience a spike in your pain with the extra activity associated with their visit.

There are many different ways in which clever planning can help you manage your pain. For example, I recently met a student who found that the two-hour drive home from university at the weekend increased her pain. As a result, she had to break up her commute by visiting friends who lived about halfway home. She knew that after about an hour of driving, her pain began to increase, so she consistently planned to meet her friends in an attempt to pace her driving activity.

I often suggest that people spend a few minutes a week, perhaps on a Sunday evening, planning their week. I have a work diary and my life is planned out many weeks in advance in that diary. While it can sometimes feel like all the spontaneity has been taken out of life, it can be very useful. It allows me to see which days are very busy. Even though I do not live with pain, I try to have days that are less demanding before or after a hectic one.

If you are not already using a diary, I think it is worth using a paper or phone diary to plan your week. A diary is useful, regardless of whether you are in paid employment or not. A diary allows you to schedule your activities; activities that are pleasurable, like meeting a friend for coffee, and less pleasurable activities, like cleaning the bathroom. It will allow you to see if there are days in the week where you have many activities planned and days in the week where you have little. You may decide to balance out your schedule by being a little more active on your 'quiet day'.

This scheduling of activity is particularly helpful if your mood is low, and I will talk more about that in my chapter on managing low mood and depression. However, even if your mood is not low, it is worth scheduling and planning your activity. The important thing to remember when you are planning and scheduling is to be flexible. I will talk about flexibility below.

Prioritising

Prioritising is another important skill to learn when you are managing your pain. Prioritising is essentially making a list, either mentally or on paper, of the things that you need to do that day, week, or month, and then working your way down the list, starting with the task that has the highest priority.

I have a busy working life, and every morning I spend a few minutes writing my list and prioritising what I want to do that day. Inevitably, some things do not get done on a particular day. This is frustrating for me, as I want to get all my tasks completed, but I have to accept that if I did complete all my tasks, I would end up working very long hours and that I would see less of my family that day, which I am rarely prepared to do.

I also need to be flexible during the day. I could plan to spend the last hour of my working day writing reports, but then a colleague can ring me to discuss a project that we are working on. This discussion could take 45 minutes, leaving very little time to finish my reports. It is easy to become stressed about such a disruption to my plan, but I recognise that flexibility is important for everyone.

Prioritising helps you to be flexible. Once you have decided on which activities are the most important to accomplish on a certain day, you often feel less stressed about not achieving those at the bottom of your priority list.

Life constantly throws curve balls at us, and some are thrown so fast that we struggle to adapt. However, if we can learn to go with the flow a little more – learn to plan, prioritise and be flexible when our plans do not work out – we will be happier. If you can learn to do this, you will be able to manage your pain better.

In my experience, people struggle with implementing the 3 Ps. I believe this is because they find it difficult to accept that they have to pace, plan, and prioritise. I also believe that the difficulty with pacing is due to the struggle with breaking the rules. When you learn to cope with being a rule-breaker, pacing, planning and prioritising become so much easier. That is when you can begin to enjoy a better quality of life!

Things to Remember

- We all have rules that we live by. Often, we are not aware that we have internalised these rules.

- Our rules can become problematic if we follow them rigidly, or if our circumstances have changed and the rules no longer serve us.

- It can be helpful to take some time out to reflect on your internalised rules, and to determine if they help you manage your pain.

- Pacing, planning, and prioritising are important pain management tools that can help you escape the boom-bust cycle of activity.

CHAPTER 6: BECOME MORE MINDFUL

> *Many people are alive but don't touch the miracle of being alive.*
> **Thich Nhat Hanh**

People are not very good at living in the present. A lot of the time, we are sleepwalking through life. Research shows that for almost 50% of the time, we are not fully present.[1] We spend a lot of time 'in our heads'; caught up in the past or the future. One of the things that distinguish us from animals is our capacity to do this.

We can remember and reflect on the past. This can be very beneficial for us. We can reflect on mistakes that we have made in the past, we can learn from them, and as a result, we can live a better life.

The ability to think about the future also serves us well. If we weren't able to spend time thinking about the future, our lives would be very chaotic. Time spent thinking about the future helps us to plan and prepare for what is to come.

While we need to spend time in the past and the future, we know that spending a lot of time in these places can be unhelpful.

Let me tell you a story to illustrate this.

I want you to imagine that on a wet and windy evening, I return home from work. I am looking forward to getting home, getting dry, sitting beside the fire for a while. When I arrive at the front door, I find it locked. I look through the window in the door and see my husband inside, making dinner. I knock on the door, see him glance over, and know that he has heard and seen me. I notice that he just ignores me and continues cooking. I knock again; he glances at me again but carries on cooking. How do you think I

---

[1] Killingsworth, M. A., & Gilbert, D. T. (2010). A Wandering Mind Is an Unhappy Mind. *Science*, 330(6006), 932–932. doi: 10.1126/science.1192439.

would feel at this point? What stories would my mind be telling me? My mind might be using some very colourful language!

I want you to imagine that 30 minutes pass before he opens the door and lets me in. What is likely to happen when I get in? Do you think that I would have anything to say to him? Am I likely to spend most of the evening thinking about it? Am I likely to bring it up again in the future?

Now, I want you to imagine something different. I want you to imagine that my dog, Charlie, is outside on a wet and windy night. He wants to get inside to lie by the fire. He goes to the front door and can see my husband cooking in the kitchen. He scrapes the front door, sees my husband glance up and notices that my husband carries on cooking. He scrapes the door a few more times, my husband glances over, shouts "in a minute Charlie" but waits until he is finished cooking, 30 minutes later, to open the door. What is Charlie's reaction when he finally gets inside? Is it different or similar to mine? Is Charlie likely to run ecstatically around the kitchen and then find a comfortable place in front of the fire? In my experience, that is exactly what he would do!

So how do Charlie and I differ in how we deal with that incident? When I get into the house, I hardly notice that I am inside; I am so angry. All I can think about is the half-hour I stood in the rain at the front door, unable to get in. That evening, all I can still think about is how my husband deliberately left me standing at the front door in the rain. The next week, I *still* think about how my husband left me standing in the rain at the front door! And Charlie, the dog, is just happy to be inside. He is in the moment; he is in the house, the heating is on, the fire is lit, and he lies in front of it to spend the evening snoozing.

This silly example illustrates the difference between humans and animals and illustrates the benefits that Charlie reaped by being in the present... by being aware that he was in the house. In this imaginary scenario, he had a much more pleasant evening than me. He didn't waste time ruminating about how awful it was to spend that time outside in the rain. While it would be ridiculous to suggest that human beings spend every minute in the present, we know that there are significant benefits associated with being more present and mindful.

The Storyteller Mind

As humans, we tend to spend a lot of time ruminating about the past; often going over and over past stories and hurts. We can get lost in these stories.

I can recall a patient, we will call him Steven, telling me that his mind felt like a washing machine on a spin, constantly turning with stories, many of them very familiar – repeats of old stories that went around and around in his mind.

We know that ruminating, or going over old stories in our minds, can greatly add to our distress. We often spend a lot of time trying to work out why we are unhappy, trying to come up with solutions to stop experiencing these difficult emotions, and trying to find ways of blocking unpleasant feelings. Unfortunately, that often makes the situation worse.

Steven, the man who described his mind as being like a washing machine on a spin, knew that he was unhappy and desperately wanted to change this. He spent a lot of time trying to figure out *why* he was thinking the way that he did, *why* his mind was always spinning out of control – ruminating about the past and worrying about the future.

Steven tended to blame himself for his inability to stop this constant contemplating and worrying. His mind told him that he shouldn't be feeling low, that he should be able to figure out a way of pulling himself out of his depression and pain. Despite his best efforts to stop his depression, to block these distressing thoughts, however, Steven found that he continued to struggle with his pain and low mood. To use the passengers on the bus metaphor again (see Chapter 3), he stopped the bus, tried to work out who was shouting and why they were doing it, and then he attempted to wrestle them off the bus. Unfortunately, he had no sooner started driving the bus again when he noticed that the unpleasant passengers were back on the bus, and that they were as vocal as ever!

Often, spending too much time reflecting on the past or thinking about the future is not helpful.

As touched upon, we know that while it is essential to spend some time thinking about the future, spending a lot of time doing so can also be unhelpful. The future can seem uncertain for all of us, and more so for people living with persistent pain. It can be anxiety-provoking to think about the future. Our minds are very good at telling us scary stories about what might happen. For example, your mind might tell you that if your pain continues like this, you will end up in a wheelchair, or your partner will get fed up and leave you.

As I said in a previous chapter, our minds tend to act like fortune tellers, making predictions about what will happen in the future. Often those predictions focus on undesirable or even catastrophic outcomes. The human mind is very good at conjuring up unpleasant stories. This, as you might remember, is because your mind tends to try to protect you from harm. By conjuring up frightening stories, or worst-case scenarios, it tries to keep you within your comfort zone, where your mind knows you are safest.

Many people have told me that since they have developed their pain, they notice that they have been spending *more and more* time thinking about the past and fretting about the future. When they think about the past, they may be thinking about old, difficult memories. Alternatively, they may be drawn to happy memories, but sometimes this can be a source of distress for them too, because they then compare their 'old life' – before they developed their pain – to their current life or their life with pain. Often, this comparison is emotionally painful and can lead to thoughts about how awful their life is now that they have persistent pain.

I can recall someone who worked as a hairdresser and had her own business. She eventually had to sell her business as she could no longer run it due to her pain. She spent a lot of time thinking about her 'old life' as a hairdresser, when she enjoyed spending time with her customers, earning a good living. She constantly compared this to her current life; when she did this, she noticed that her mood lowered.

I also remember another patient who managed to stay in work despite his pain. He spent a lot of time worrying about the future, how he would manage his heavy workload given his persistent pain. He noticed that these worrying thoughts had a negative impact on his emotional wellbeing and his pain.

What Can We Do About This?

Practising mindfulness can help counter the impact of our negative thinking. Meditation is a great way to practise mindfulness, but there is more to mindfulness than just meditation, as I will explain below.

Mindfulness is trendy these days; it pops up all the time in newspapers, magazines, and online articles. You would be forgiven for thinking that mindfulness is a new 'discovery' but, in fact, it is thousands of years old.

What is Mindfulness?

Dr Jon Kabat-Zinn[2] defines mindfulness as "Awareness that arises through paying attention, on purpose, in the present moment, non-judgementally."

Let's break this down a little more.

"Awareness that arises through paying attention" means noticing or becoming aware. As we have already discovered, much of what goes on in our minds does so without us being aware of it. Our minds are constantly chattering; sometimes we may be aware of it, but at other times we are in 'autopilot mode' or unaware of what is going on. "On purpose" means deliberately attempting to notice and become aware. "In the present moment" means what is going on right here, right now, in this second. "Non-judgementally" means just what it says, without assessment. It is my experience that the "non-judgemental" part of mindfulness can be particularly tricky for people who live with pain.

---

[2] Kabat-Zinn, J. (2005). *Wherever you go, there you are: mindfulness meditation in everyday life*. New York: Hachette Books.

As I have mentioned a few times, I have noticed that people who live with persistent pain can become very critical and judgemental not of others, but of themselves.

Let's consider Steven's situation again, and his concerns about his 'washing machine mind'. He began to notice what was going on in his mind – the stories that his mind was telling him, the emotions that he was feeling. He was very critical about what he was noticing – constantly berating himself for having these thoughts and experiencing these emotions. He told himself that he had no right to feel depressed, that he had a home and a lovely wife and family. This judgemental attitude further escalated his suffering and added significantly to his distress.

The Benefits of Mindfulness

There is a growing scientific evidence base about the benefits of mindfulness in health generally, and the field of pain management specifically. Mindfulness training has been linked to lower stress levels. People who regularly practise mindfulness meditation are happier and more contented than the average person. Regular mindfulness meditation can reduce anxiety, depression, and irritability.

It has been shown that being mindful of our emotions helps us to adopt a more positive mindset. People who practise mindfulness often report improved relationships with others. It has also been shown that practising mindfulness can help us sleep better.

Amazingly, studies have shown that practising mindfulness meditation helps the immune system, and that people who meditate regularly are better at fighting off simple illnesses like colds, as well as more serious health conditions.

As I said a moment ago, you would be forgiven for thinking that mindfulness meditation is a new phenomenon; it seems very in vogue now. However, we know that meditation is an ancient practice. What is new, though, is our ability to see how it changes the brain. We now have access to wonderful technology, functional magnetic resonance imaging (fMRI). You may be familiar with this technology (maybe you even had an MRI to help your doctor make a diagnosis concerning your pain). fMRIs take pictures of the brain and also record brain activity during the scan. Research using fMRIs has shown us that people who meditate regularly experience changes in the part of the brain called the amygdala, which is considered to be the 'fight or flight' centre of the brain. It is associated with fear and emotion, and it is involved in the body's stress response.[3] This finding is particularly important for people who live with pain, as we know that stress can make persistent pain worse.

Mindfulness Meditation and Persistent Pain

When we consider persistent pain, we understand that it is entirely normal to want it just to stop, to go away permanently. When you think about mindfulness, you may be concerned that if you become more mindful, then you are going to become even more aware of your pain and notice it even more.

It may seem counterintuitive, but becoming more aware of what is going on in your body, and what is going on in your mind, does help you to manage persistent pain better. For example, a research paper from 2018[4] found that mindfulness-based meditation lowered the perception of pain, increased mobility, and improved functioning and well-being among people living with persistent pain. The researchers concluded that mindfulness-based interventions should be utilised in pain clinics and that clinicians using these interventions could potentially help improve treatment outcomes and help their patients to reduce their medication use.

---

[3] Taren, A. A., Creswell, J. D., & Gianaros, P. J. (2013). Dispositional Mindfulness Co-Varies with Smaller Amygdala and Caudate Volumes in Community Adults. *PLoS ONE*, 8(5). doi: 10.1371/journal.pone.0064574.

[4] Majeed, M. H., Ali, A. A., & Sudak, D. M. (2018). Mindfulness-based interventions for chronic pain: Evidence and applications. *Asian Journal of Psychiatry*, 32, 79–83. doi: 10.1016/j.ajp.2017.11.025.

What is Mindfulness Meditation?

When I discuss mindfulness meditation with people, I often find that they say things like, "I can't do it, I can't focus, I can't empty my mind." I always reply that it is entirely normal for your mind to wander when you are meditating. There is a real misconception that meditation is emptying your mind!

> **Mindfulness meditation is not about emptying your mind – it is about noticing what is going on in your mind.**

My own experience of meditation has taught me that some days when I meditate, my mind is fairly 'quiet'; on other days, my mind is all over the place – jumping from thought to thought, from a thought to an emotion, and back to a thought again. Having sat there peacefully – while I noticed my mind flitting about – does not mean that I did not meditate that day, or that I failed in my meditation, or did it wrong; it just means that I had a different experience when meditating and that is ok. That is still meditation.

An easy way to begin to understand mindfulness meditation is to imagine that you are sitting at the side of the road watching the traffic go by. There is a steady stream of traffic: big vans, noisy smelly lorries, old back-firing cars, shiny sleek cars, and so on. Your only job is to sit and notice them. At no time are you expected to walk out into the middle of the road, to stop the traffic or tell the noisy, smelly lorries that they need to take a different route.

As we meditate, we become the observer of the traffic in our mind. All of us have thoughts and experience emotions that are pleasant. We also experience thoughts and emotions that are not so pleasant. It is really important to appreciate that these thoughts and emotions are transient; like the traffic on the road, they come and they go.

To illustrate this point, try this exercise. Recall a time when you were ecstatic with happiness. It may be the day your child was born, or the day that you got married, or the day that you got divorced! Either way, did that feeling of ecstatic happiness last? No, it didn't. It passed.

Think of another strong emotion that you experienced. Perhaps, an intense feeling of disappointment. Maybe you didn't get that job that you wanted. Perhaps you weren't able to buy or rent that house that you loved. Did that feeling persist? No, it didn't. You may have felt disappointed for some time but, eventually, that feeling passed as well.

We often get caught up in the belief that our current situation is awful, that it is unbearable, that it will never end. One of my favourite sayings is, "This too will pass". Mindfulness meditation helps remind us that everything in our minds is transient; thoughts and emotions pass, just like the noisy lorries and the sleek soft-top sports car on the imaginary road described above.

How Can Mindfulness Meditation Change How We Relate to Our Emotions?

It is normal for us to experience different emotions, like surprise, sadness, anger, fear, disgust, joy, and so on. How we relate to those normal emotional fluctuations can add to our distress, or can provide us with a sense of awareness about ourselves that can support us in our daily lives.

I want you to imagine someone who has struggled with anxiety. I want you to consider how they might think if they notice that they are feeling anxious for no apparent reason. They are not aware of any particular trigger for the anxiety; they just notice that they are feeling anxious. What might happen if this person frantically tries to discover the trigger for their anxiety? What if they have the thought, "Oh no, my anxiety is out of control, I have nothing to feel anxious about but my stomach is churning with anxiety"? What might happen?

It is very likely that a person who experiences such thoughts will feel *anxious about their anxiety* and that this will make their distress even worse.

What about an alternative way of being?

Imagine this: the person notices that she feels anxious, but recognises it as a transient emotion, something that is present but which will pass, just like those noisy lorries on the road. Research evidence suggests that this 'mindful awareness of anxious feelings' is helpful; people who often experience anxiety about their anxiety find that their suffering decreases as a result of mindfulness.

As well as helping us appreciate that our thoughts and emotions are temporary, mindfulness meditation can help us choose *how* we want to behave or act.

For example, if this person has been practising mindfulness meditation for a while, she might notice that she has got caught in a series of thoughts or stories about herself. She may be able to take a step back from them and make decisions about what to do based on her values, rather than the directions and stories that her mind has generated.

Become an Observer of Your Mind

I was recently talking with Susan, who had lost confidence since she developed her pain. She had become very anxious about driving. Susan continued to drive short, local journeys, but she had been avoiding longer journeys. She identified that this was having a negative impact on her life and that her independence had been affected.

Susan was aware that every time she contemplated going on a long journey, she experienced anxiety and had thoughts like, "You are not a good driver, you are likely to get into an accident if you try this longer drive." By developing the ability to take a step back from her thoughts through meditation, and by developing the capacity to notice that she was dwelling on a frightening imagined future event, Susan was able to recognise that she had two choices: 1. she could act on her negative thoughts and avoid driving longer journeys, or 2. do something different; try to gradually increase the distance that she drove.

Susan was able to recognise that she valued being independent and she decided that she wanted to move towards this value by continuing to drive her car, despite her anxiety. She allowed her behaviour to be influenced by her values and not the frightening stories that her mind told her.

You will remember that I told you about Viktor Frankl in Chapter 2. When I consider the freedom that comes from recognising that our thoughts do not have to control our behaviour, I am reminded of the following quote by Dr Frankl:

> **Between stimulus and response, there is a space. In that space is our power to choose our response. In our response lies our growth and our freedom.**

How Do You Begin to Practise Mindfulness Meditation, and How Do You Become More Mindful?

Let's start with mindfulness meditation. Very simply, this involves taking some time out to just notice what is going on in your mind. It can be done anywhere, at any time, but I think it is easiest to start your practice at home in an area where you will not be disturbed. I remember when I first started meditating, I asked my children not to disturb me as I wanted to meditate. The first few times I asked them this, they rolled their eyes at me and called me a hippy. They presumed I would be sitting crossed-legged on the floor making peace signs.

Meditation does not have to involve sitting cross-legged, wearing a bandana or a sarong. If you are comfortable sitting cross-legged, by all means, do that. However, it is often recommended that people meditate sitting in a comfortable chair where you can maintain an upright position without any significant discomfort. People often ask me about meditating in bed. You can do that if it is your most comfortable position. However, meditation is an active practice, and if possible, it is best to practise outside of your bed, at least some of the time. It is also best if you can try and find somewhere to meditate where you will be undisturbed, where the dog won't be jumping on you, the phone won't be ringing, or the children won't be asking you, "What's for dinner?" You do not need to find a perfectly quiet place to meditate. When I meditate at home, I can hear background traffic noise and the sounds of my family getting on with their lives. That background noise is fine; it just drifts in and out of my awareness. It is best to have your legs and arms uncrossed when you are sitting in your chair meditating. You can rest your hands gently on your lap if that feels comfortable to you.

People are often unsure how long to meditate for. There is a misconception that you have to do it for long periods every day, to experience any benefits of meditation.

A lot of people find that a 10-minute daily practice is a good starting point. When people have got used to incorporating this 10-minute daily meditation practice into their day, they sometimes want to increase the time that they spend meditating. Other people remain with a 10-minute daily practice.

Meditation is a skill, and as such it tends to develop with regular practice. Try to practise daily. If this is not possible for you, just try to practise as regularly as possible.

It is helpful to meditate with your eyes closed. If that feels uncomfortable to you, you can find a spot on the floor to direct your focus. When you initially sit down to meditate, you might choose to spend a few seconds noticing how your body feels on the chair, the parts of your body that are touching the chair. You could notice how your hands feel in your lap and how your feet feel on the floor.

When you start to practise mindfulness meditation, it is useful to use your breath as an anchor or a focus. You are always breathing; your breath is always with you. Therefore, your breath is available to use as an anchor 24/7, any time, any place. What this means is just becoming aware of your breath, not trying to practise deep breathing or change your breathing in any way; just resting your awareness on your breath. Just noticing the sensations of your breathing.

Some people find it helpful to count their breaths, especially when they are learning to practise mindfulness meditation. If you want to try this, you can start by counting 1 as you breathe in, and 2 as you breathe out, then 3 when you next breathe in, and 4 as you breathe out again, and so on up to 10. When you get to 10, you can start at 1 again. If you get lost or distracted and do not know what number you are on, don't worry, just start at 1 again.

As you are counting your breaths, you will get distracted. Thoughts will come into your head, perhaps things like "This is a waste of time," or "My back is so sore today," or "I am looking forward to my dinner tonight," or "I should have gone to the bathroom before I started this," or "What is the dog barking at?" or "I am so fed up today." Your only task when you notice that you have become distracted is to bring your attention back to your breath.

You are likely to be distracted by your mind many times during a short meditation practice. This is a normal mind at work, so there is no need to give yourself a hard time – remember, one of the core aspects of mindfulness meditation is about being non-judgemental in your practice. You can just notice where your mind has gone and re-direct your attention back to your breath.

At the end of your meditation practice, it can be helpful to spend a couple of seconds with your eyes closed, just resting. You can then ground yourself back in the present by noticing again how your body feels on the chair, how your feet feel on the floor, and noticing any sounds that you can hear.

People often notice that they feel more relaxed and calmer after meditating. However, that is not always the case, and if you do not experience any feelings of relaxation, it doesn't mean that you have done anything wrong or that you cannot meditate.

I have summarised the steps for meditating in the exercise below.

Steps for Practising Mindfulness Meditation

Sit in a comfortable upright chair with your feet flat on the floor. If that is too uncomfortable for you, due to your pain, find a comfortable position that helps you remain awake and aware.

Close your eyes. If that doesn't feel comfortable find a spot on the floor to gently focus on.

Spend a couple of minutes noticing the part of your body that is in contact with the chair; notice how your hands feel resting in your lap and how your feet feel on the floor.

Move your focus to your breath. Notice where – in your body – you feel the breath the most; it may be your stomach, chest, nose or mouth. Do not try to change your breath. Just notice how it feels to breathe normally.

If it is helpful, begin to count the breaths, the first inhale as 1, the exhale as 2, and so on, up to 10. Start again at 1 and continue doing this for a few minutes.

Your mind is likely to wander. When you notice this, bring your attention gently back to the breath. There is no need to give yourself a hard time about this. Just notice that your attention has wandered and bring your attention back to the breath.

Continue to focus on your breath and when you notice your mind has been pulled away, gently bring it back to the breath without judgement.

Finish your practice by moving your focus from your breath back to how your body feels on the chair, how your feet feel on the floor. Notice any sounds that you hear.

Open your eyes and bring your attention back to the room.

Resources

There are some great resources online that can help you begin your mindfulness practice. Many people find 'guided meditations' beneficial; these are audio recordings in which somebody talks you through what you need to do and what you could focus on – all you have to do is listen and follow the instructions. I used guided meditations to help me start my practice, and I continue to use them today, as I find them so valuable. There are many websites and phone apps which provide guided mindfulness meditations that allow you to develop and move forward with your practice. [5] In turn, many websites or apps offer taster sessions for free, and if you find a particular one useful, you can often subscribe for access to more sessions or recordings. Many of these sessions are

---

[5] I find the website www.headspace.com particularly useful, but there are many others.

focused on particular difficulties – for example, sleep and anxiety – and some also have sessions specifically focused on pain.

Becoming More Mindful in Your Daily Life

When you regularly engage in formal meditation practices like the one described above, you may notice that you will become more mindful in your day-to-day life. You might become more aware of when your 'washing machine mind' is on a spin, and you will develop a greater awareness of the chatter in your mind.

With this increased awareness of your mind's talk, you will probably be able to recognise when your mind is repeating old unhelpful stories about the past or frightening, worrying stories about the future. Through this awareness, you will develop the capacity to bring your mind back to the present when this is helpful for you.

Gradually, you may become aware that going over old stuff in your head, or worrying about the future and running through possible scenarios of how things might go wrong, is a terrible waste of your time. You might realise how many times stories have taken over your mind. There is a saying that you "don't have to listen to the rumours in your mind" but how often have you done just that and got caught up in all the projections of your brain? Do you ever ask yourself if that time is well spent? Maybe it would have been more enjoyable if you had been able to just live in the moment.

Have you ever been on a car or train journey when you realised that you were almost at your destination and that you were so lost in thought you hadn't even noticed the places that you were travelling through? Perhaps you were so lost in your thoughts that you forgot to get off the bus at the right place.

We all tend to get lost in our heads; we are present but not really 'present'. When you practise mindfulness meditation, you get more skilled at noticing when you are not present and you can bring yourself back to the only moment you have, the 'now'.

Daily Mindful Practices

Being mindful is not just about starting a formal mindfulness meditation. You can practise being mindful by taking a few moments, or minutes, to consciously increase your awareness of the here and now and all that is around you. There are several mindful practices that you can do anywhere – at home, at work, in the car, or standing in a queue in a shop. You could practise mindfulness when you are doing the most mundane of tasks. For example, you could practise mindfulness when you are brushing your teeth; noticing the sound of the water, the taste of the toothpaste, the feel of the toothbrush on your teeth.

I have suggested a few brief mindful practices below that you might find useful to incorporate into your everyday life.

Noticing

3-2-1 noticing exercise

Notice 3 things that you can see, hear, and feel.

Notice 2 things that you can see, hear, and feel

Notice 1 thing that you can see, hear, and feel

With this exercise, you start by noticing three things that you can see, hear and feel, then two things, and so on.

For example, if I practise this now...

- I can see my pen on the table, I can see the cream curtains, and I can see a green field through the window.

- I can hear a dog barking, I can hear birds chirping, and I can hear a clock ticking.

- I can feel my watch on my arm, I can feel my feet in my shoes, and I can feel my collar on my neck.

To complete this exercise, I would then go on to notice two things and finally one thing in each of the three categories (see, hear, feel).

Don't worry if you can't notice enough things to complete the exercise. For example, if you are in a quiet environment, it might be hard to notice things that you can hear. This exercise is just about bringing your awareness to the present. You don't have to complete it, as described above, every time.

Mindful Breaths

Bring your focus to your breath.

Notice the inhale and the exhale.

Follow this for three breaths or as many as you like.

Mindful Walking

If you want to practise mindful walking, you can choose to notice what you are doing and what is happening when you are on foot, instead of letting your mind wander. You can notice how each step feels as you put your foot to the ground, you can notice how the breeze feels on your face, how the sun feels on your arms. You can tune into the sounds that you hear, perhaps the sound of the wind rustling through the trees, the birds singing, or the sounds of the cars passing by on the road. Essentially, you are gently focusing your mind on the present, rather than letting it wander into the past or future.

Mindful Eating

How many times have you eaten something and realised that you hadn't even tasted it? You may have been watching TV and went to take another crisp when you noticed the bag was empty? Perhaps you were driving the car and went to take another sweet and realised that you had finished them all without even really being aware that you were eating them? We know that we do many things *mindlessly,* and eating is also one of them. Mindful eating may help people who have trouble maintaining a healthy weight, as we know that we can reduce our tendency to overeat if we eat mindfully. It can be helpful to try a mindful eating practice to see what your experience is.

In introductory mindfulness courses, people are typically asked to practise mindful eating with raisins. I have outlined the steps below, and I have chosen to use chocolate as an example because of own my tendency towards mindless chocolate eating, but if you want, you can choose to substitute the chocolate for a raisin or other food substance.

Mindful Chocolate Eating

Sit somewhere quiet where you will not be disturbed. Turn off the TV and the radio and focus on this task only.

Open a chocolate bar and take your time to examine a piece of it. Look at it like you have never seen chocolate before; look at the colour and feel the texture.

Put a piece of chocolate in your mouth and let it sit on your tongue.

Notice the texture and flavour. Notice the urge to bite into it.

Allow the chocolate to melt into your mouth. Swallow the melted chocolate.

When you have eaten this piece of chocolate, break off the next piece and repeat the steps above.

Finally, notice what was different about the experience when you compare it to your usual way of eating chocolate.

I wanted to include the mindful eating exercise because many people have told me that they comfort eat in an attempt to get some relief from their pain. I can appreciate why they do it; when you are in pain, you will often take any comfort that you can get. I think there are very few people in the world that do not engage in emotional eating, whether they live with pain or not.

People engage in emotional eating for many reasons; they may eat to cope with stress, low mood, loneliness, or simply because they are bored. If you are someone who tends to engage in emotional eating, you might consider incorporating this practice into your day. Of course, it is ridiculous to suggest that you would eat like this all the time, but I think that an occasional practice of mindful eating would be useful to help you recognise when you are eating mindlessly and to support you in becoming more mindful when you are eating. You will find more tips on managing emotional eating in Chapter 12.

In summary, we know that humans tend to get excessively caught up in the past and the future, and in doing so, lose contact with the present. Practising mindfulness has many benefits and could be a helpful tool for you in your pain management toolbox.

Things to Remember

- Most of us spend a lot of time caught up 'in our heads'. We are not good at living in the present and noticing what is going on inside us and in the world around us.

- Many of us spend time ruminating; repeating old stories from the past or worrying about the future.

- Practising mindfulness can help us notice how our thoughts are driving our emotions and behaviour.

- Research has found that people who regularly practise mindfulness live happier lives.

- Studies have also shown that practising mindfulness meditation can help with pain management.

CHAPTER 7: UNDERSTAND STRESS AND ANXIETY

> *Our anxiety does not come from thinking about the future, but from wanting to control it.*
>
> **Kahlil Gibran**

I have dedicated this chapter to exploring anxiety and stress. I know that anxiety and stress present significant difficulties for a large number of people, whether they live with pain or not. In this chapter, you will learn about the nature of anxiety and stress and – in Chapter 8 – I will share strategies that will help you manage your stress and anxiety. Please read this chapter on understanding stress and anxiety before rushing to unearth solutions; often, you will find that understanding a problem contributes to your management of its symptoms.

The terms stress and anxiety are often used interchangeably. However, there is a difference between them. Stress, unlike anxiety, is a response to the pressures that we feel in life, to the stressors that we encounter. When we experience stress for a long time, we can develop other difficulties like depression and anxiety. Though anxiety and stress are closely related, not all people who experience stress will develop difficulties with anxiety.

I think that it is impossible to go through life without experiencing some stressful situations. If you are alive and breathing, you are going to encounter stressors. These stressors may just be everyday hassles, like trying to find your child's missing school shoe when he is already late for school, or having to deal with traffic jams on the way to work, or trying to find a parking place at the hospital when you are late for your appointment.

While I have dedicated this chapter and Chapter 8 to the discussion of anxiety, and to provide you with some tips and techniques that will help you manage it, the anxiety management techniques outlined will also help you manage stress.

> **Even if you don't experience any difficulties when managing anxiety and stress, it is still worth reading these next two chapters and trying to incorporate some of the techniques described into your life.**

What is Anxiety?

Anxiety is known to be a major mental health problem. Let's spend a few moments talking about mental health.

When I consider mental health, I find it helpful to think about your mental health as being on a continuum. Just like your physical health, there will be times in your life when your mental health is better than other times. If you experience a difficult time in your life, for example, if you have a family bereavement of if you are having a very stressful time at work, your mental health may deteriorate somewhat. At other times in your life, your mental health may improve. As a psychologist, I think it is essential that everyone learns some basic skills to help them maintain good mental health, and to help them improve their mental health when it is poor.

Research indicates that approximately 1 in 4 people in the UK will experience a mental health problem in any one year[6]. A recently published survey that was carried out in England found that the most common mental health problems experienced by people are generalised anxiety disorder followed by depression[7]. If your mental health is currently poor you are not alone. The good news is that there are many things that you can do to help improve it.

---

[6] McManus, S., Meltzer, H., Brugha, T. S., Bebbington, P. E., & Jenkins, R. (2009). *Adult psychiatric morbidity in England, 2007: results of a household survey.* The NHS Information Centre for health and social care.

[7] McManus S, Bebbington P, Jenkins R, Brugha T. (eds.) (2016). *Mental health and wellbeing in England: Adult psychiatric morbidity survey 2014.* Leeds: NHS digital.

Anxiety is normal, we all experience a certain level of anxiety at times. Anxiety is a customary response to situations that we see as threatening to us. One dictionary definition describes the word anxiety as "an uncomfortable feeling of nervousness or worry about something that is happening or might happen in the future."[8] It is not 'a bad emotion'.

Anxiety can be helpful; we know that anxiety can help us perform better or cope in an emergency. If humans did not experience anxiety, the human race would probably have joined the dinosaurs in extinction. Imagine if our ancestors could not experience anxiety; there would be nothing to prevent them from deciding to pet the lion's beautiful golden mane!

However, for some people anxiety can become problematic. People may fail to notice, at first, that anxiety has become a difficulty for them. Many patients have told me that before the development of their pain, they would never have regarded themselves as 'an anxious person', and they are surprised that anxiety has become part of their lives now.

When you experience a lot of anxiety, it can be associated with some unpleasant physical symptoms. These symptoms can be frightening, particularly if you don't know why you are experiencing them, or if you believe that these symptoms are a sign that there is something seriously wrong with you.

The worry about being overwhelmed with anxiety can stop people from doing things that they want to do, and from doing things that are important to them. Patients have told me that their anxiety stops them from going to important family events such as weddings and birthday parties, that it stops them from going shopping or out for a meal, and that it stops them from attending other important events like parent-teacher meetings.

Anxiety affects us in at least four different ways. It affects our body and we may experience physical symptoms. It affects the way that we think, it affects the way that we feel, and it also affects the way that we behave. Let's look at each of those categories in turn.

---

[8] Cambridge dictionary online.

Anxiety may Affect your Body

- Your heart may race, pound, or skip a beat.

- Your chest may feel tight or painful.

- You may notice that you have to go to the toilet more frequently.

- Your breathing will change; you may notice that your breathing has become faster and shallow.

- You may feel dizzy and light-headed.

- You may notice that you are sweating more than normal.

- Your muscles may feel tense and your body may ache more than normal.

- You may notice butterflies in your stomach or that your stomach is churning.

- Your mouth may become dry.

- You may feel jumpy or restless, like you have to keep moving.

- You might feel tingling or numbness in your fingers and toes.

Anxiety may Affect How you Think

People who have difficulties with anxiety often report the following symptoms:

- I am always worrying.

- I go over the same worrying thoughts over and over again.

- I imagine the worst and think about it a lot of the time.

- I find it difficult to concentrate.

- My thoughts race.

I have listed a few examples of worrying thoughts that someone who has difficulties with anxiety may notice.

- I am going to lose control and make a fool of myself in front of everyone.

- My heart is racing so bad. I must be having a heart attack.

- I am not going to be able to manage the stairs and find the bathrooms.

- The doctors have missed something, I am seriously ill.

- People will see me using my crutch and think that I am trying to appear worse than I am.

- I have a feeling something awful is going to happen.

- I am going to faint.

Anxiety may Affect How you Feel

- You may feel worried, nervous, tense, and frightened.

- You may feel as if you are not really in your body.

- You may feel panicky and woozy.

Anxiety may Affect your Behaviour

- You may find it difficult to sit still and you may have to move, fidget, or pace up and down.

- You may find it hard to relax.

- You may notice that your speech is faster than normal.

- You may feel more irritable than normal, and you may tend to snap at others.

- You may drink and/or smoke more than usual to cope with these unpleasant symptoms.

- You may avoid things that make you anxious.

What is the Function of Anxiety?

As I wrote above, anxiety – like fear – can be useful. It helps to keep us safe. Many years ago, the world was a very dangerous place. Resources like food were limited and people had to fight for the things that we needed to survive. We developed the capacity to feel anxious to keep safe in this dangerous world. When we encountered physical danger, like a wild animal or our neighbour trying to steal our steak, we had three options – *freeze, fight, or flight*.

We know that the 'freeze, fight, or flight' response was vital to human survival back then.

We have a better chance of escaping danger if our body is pumped up for it. Anxiety makes us alert, tense, and ready to deal with the danger that we have encountered. When we experience anxiety, we might notice that:

- Our hearts begin beating more quickly (supplying blood to our muscles).

- We sweat (to cool us down).

- Our muscles become tense (ready for action).

- We take deeper breaths (to supply oxygen to our muscles).

In essence, all of these responses are supposed to aid our escape or improve our ability to stay and fight the danger. When considered in this way, we can see how the symptoms of anxiety are beneficial. Indeed, all of the physical symptoms we experience, when anxious, played a helpful role in protecting us in dangerous pre-historic circumstances.

Thankfully, the world has moved on and most of us are lucky enough to live in a physically safe environment where we don't have to fight over food or shelter, or wrestle and kill wild animals to survive. However, the human brain is still very good at scanning the environment and trying to detect danger, even if that danger is not the kind of danger that you can fight or run from.

In modern times, the danger or threat can take many other forms like:

- I won't be able to pay the mortgage this month.

- I don't think my partner finds me attractive any more.

- My doctor doesn't believe that my pain is real.

- My son should have been home hours ago; I think he has had an accident.

- My pain is getting worse and worse. Soon I am not going to be able to continue with my job.

- I am going to become so disabled that I will end up in a wheelchair.

> **It is important to remember that the symptoms of too much anxiety are very unpleasant but they are not dangerous.**

Remembering that anxiety symptoms are unpleasant but not dangerous can help you become less fearful of them; this will allow them to pass sooner.

Anxiety symptoms can be very nasty and when you are already in pain, they can become even more unpleasant and frightening. Many patients have told me that it has been helpful to realise that these unpleasant symptoms are normal responses to threat and danger. We all need to remember that it is commonplace to feel anxiety and everyone experiences it.

However, it can be useful to work out if anxiety has become a difficulty for you. In some cases, we may speak of 'an anxiety disorder', when levels of anxiety are so high that they can affect a person's daily life. If the following apply to you, it may be the case that anxiety has become problematic for you:

- The symptoms of anxiety are very severe and unpleasant.

- You are experiencing these symptoms very frequently.

- These symptoms persist for a long time when they occur.

- These symptoms are causing you to worry that there is something seriously wrong with you.

- Anxiety is stopping you from doing things that you want to do.

Causes of Anxiety

Many different factors can lead to someone having difficulties with anxiety. If people have had difficult experiences when they were younger, they may notice that they feel anxious a lot of the time. Nobody escapes experiencing stressful life events, like illness, bereavements, divorce, or financial difficulties. All of these life events and stressors can contribute towards someone developing difficulties with anxiety.

Occupational stress can also cause people to develop difficulties with anxiety; working long hours, an unsupportive boss, and/or difficult colleagues can contribute towards the development of anxiety difficulties. Relationship or family problems may also be a factor.

Without doubt, living with persistent pain is also a *very significant* stressor that can contribute towards the development of difficulties with anxiety.

Some people can't identify any particular cause for their anxiety. There doesn't have to be any single reason for problems for anxiety to develop, and sometimes psychologists use a bucket metaphor to explain the development of anxiety difficulties.

Imagine that you have a bucket that is filling up with stressor after stressor; lack of sleep due to pain, difficulty managing workload due to pain, financial difficulties, noisy neighbours. It won't be long until that bucket starts to overfill. Subsequently, it might be one relatively small stressor that causes the bucket to overflow and for anxiety difficulties to develop. We need to find ways of emptying some of the water from the bucket. There are many stress and anxiety management techniques that have been developed that will help you do that. I will describe these techniques in the next chapter (Chapter 8).

When people develop difficulties with anxiety, they try to cope as best they can. Some of the things they do are helpful, but sometimes their actions are only helpful in the short-term; over the long-term, they only add to the problem. For example, sometimes people drink more than is healthy in an attempt to relax. People can also use drugs to cope with stress and anxiety. They can withdraw from their friends and family, spend many hours binge-watching boxsets on TV, and do other things that are ultimately unhelpful – no matter how good they make them feel at the time.

Thoughts about Symptoms of Anxiety

How people *think* about and *interpret* their symptoms can also *add* to their anxiety. Consider the physical symptoms above. Are any of them symptomatic of a potentially life-threatening condition? A racing heart, pain in the chest? I don't think it is unreasonable for someone who is experiencing such symptoms to assume that they are having a heart attack.

What would happen to your anxiety levels if you thought that you were having a heart attack? Mine would go sky high! The difficulty with these symptoms is they are so real and unpleasant that it is easy to interpret them as a sign of something very sinister. This interpretation causes a massive surge in anxiety, which in turn causes these symptoms, and so we enter a vicious cycle of anxiety.

One way of breaking the vicious cycle is to understand the symptoms of anxiety and remember that they are essentially your body in 'fight or flight mode'. As mentioned above, they are caused by your brain trying to do a good job in keeping you safe.

Avoidance

Another factor that can maintain an individual's difficulties with anxiety is avoidance. We have talked about this in a previous chapter but it is worth mentioning again here. We avoid what scares us, it is human nature. As I explained previously, avoidance is not a problem if we avoid things that do not have a big impact on our lives. If spiders make us anxious, and we avoid them as a result, it is no big deal provided we can persuade someone else to deal with them for us. However, what happens if you have started avoiding some of the important things in life?

Let's consider Emma's experience. Emma was in her 30s and was embarrassed that she walked slowly and had to use a stick. She had begun to avoid social situations as she felt anxious when she thought that other people were looking at her (and thinking negatively about the fact that she needed to use a stick). She had noticed that the more she avoided anxiety-provoking situations, the more reluctant she became to leave her home. In the last couple of years, Emma had started avoiding parent-teacher meetings due to her anxiety. She valued her children getting a good education and she believed that – as their mother – she played a vital role in supporting them in school. Therefore, it was very distressing for her to have to ask her partner to attend the parent-teacher meetings on his own.

When I explored the situation with Emma, it was clear that she was motivated to manage her anxiety more effectively. She had clarified her values and understood that her anxiety was causing her to make choices (avoid parent-teacher meetings) that moved her away from them.

Reflecting on your values is one of the key first steps to overcoming anxiety. If you know *why* you want to overcome anxiety, you can start working towards your goal.

Emma could easily identify her 'why' when she thought about working on managing her anxiety. She knew that she wanted to be able to attend her children's parent-teacher meetings because she valued education and attending these meetings allowed her to support her children in a way that was important to her. Identifying her reasons to change was the first step for Emma but it wasn't easy for her to change her behaviour. It took time and a lot of effort for Emma to overcome her avoidance and to leave the safety of her home where she did not feel judged. Repeatedly *tuning into her values* was one of the key techniques that Emma used to overcome her difficulty with avoidance. It helped her move forward when she reminded herself *why* she was working on her avoidance.

I believe that your first step in managing anxiety is identifying your 'why'. Avoidance is very powerful and tackling avoidance is difficult, but the rewards can be great. I will talk about working with avoidance in more detail later.

A Word about Panic Attacks

It is not uncommon for people who live with persistent pain to develop panic attacks. Panic attacks can be incredibly frightening. You may feel sick during them, you may feel like you can't breathe, your heart might be racing so fast that you are convinced that you are having a heart attack, you may feel like you are going to choke to death, you may experience a ringing in your ears, you may feel that you are not really in your body (this is known as dissociation). You may also have the overwhelming desire to escape your environment. Panic attacks do not only occur during the day. People can also have a panic attack when they are sleeping and many people have told me that they have woken up sweating, feeling like that they are going to choke to death.

Some people are aware of *triggers* for their panic attacks. However, for many people, panic attacks seem to come out of the blue, for no apparent reason. This can be particularly scary as the person experiencing the panic attacks might worry that one could occur at any moment, and this makes them feel like they have no control over them. People often begin to avoid situations or events that they believe may trigger a panic attack. As you would expect, this avoidance can have a significant impact on a person's quality of life.

What is a Panic Attack?

A panic attack is a rush of intense anxiety, and the person having the panic attack experiences intense and alarming physical symptoms like those described above. Panic attacks usually last for anything from a few minutes to about twenty minutes. Most people have panic attacks very infrequently, while other people can have several panic attacks in one day. When this happens, it can seem like the panic attack has gone on for hours.

It is important to remember that although having a panic attack is a deeply unpleasant experience; panic attacks are not dangerous. The physical sensations are caused by your body going into fight or flight mode.

To rule out any underlying physical cause for your panic attacks, you could consult with your GP or doctor, especially if you believe that you still have a rapid or irregular heartbeat or chest pains after your panic attack.

Anxiety and Persistent Pain

It is not surprising that people who live with persistent pain often have difficulties with anxiety. As a result of reading the information in this book, you will know that our brain interprets pain as a signal of impending danger. Pain and anxiety both suggest that the individual who is experiencing them must take some form of action to keep safe and/or survive.

Studies on pain and anxiety suggest that anxiety amplifies the perception of pain and therefore makes the pain worse.[9] There is also growing evidence that anxiety may be inflammatory and that as a result, it *contributes* to our pain experience. It is believed that people who suffer from chronic pain and have an anxiety disorder may have a lower tolerance for pain. People with an anxiety disorder may be more sensitive to the side effects of medication, or more fearful of side effects of pain medication than somebody who doesn't have an anxiety disorder. Also, they may be more fearful of pain than someone who experiences pain without anxiety.

Now that you have learned a little more about anxiety and its relationship with pain, we can consider ways to manage it. The next chapter will provide you with practical strategies that you can implement straight away to help you manage anxiety and stress.

Things to Remember

- Anxiety is normal – we all experience anxiety at times.

- For some people, anxiety can become problematic. If they experience it frequently and/or severely, it can have a negative impact on their lives.

- Anxiety affects your body and how you think, feel, and behave.

- We often avoid things that make us anxious. This avoidance helps us reduce our anxiety in the short-term. However, it has been shown that avoidance of anxiety-provoking situations can make anxiety worse in the longer term.

- Research shows that anxiety makes pain worse.

---

[9] Rhudy, J.L., & Meagher, M.W. (2000). Fear and anxiety: divergent effects on human pain thresholds. *Pain*, 84, 65-75.

CHAPTER 8: TECHNIQUES FOR MANAGING ANXIETY AND STRESS

> *You can't stop the waves, but you can learn to surf.*
> **Jon Kabat-Zinn**

As I mentioned at the beginning of Chapter 7, there is a lot to learn about anxiety. Here, in Chapter 8, I outline some techniques for managing anxiety.

> **Remember, these techniques are also helpful for managing stress and for helping you maintain good mental health. It is worth incorporating at least some of them into your life, even if you are not currently experiencing difficulties with anxiety.**

Understand More About Anxiety

If you understand that the unpleasant symptoms of anxiety are not dangerous, harmful, or a sign that something awful is going to happen, you will have taken the first step towards managing your anxiety. If you understand that these symptoms are caused by your brain's attempts to help and protect you, you are likely to feel less anxious about the symptoms.

Learn how to Work with your Thoughts and Manage the Stories in your Mind

We have talked quite a bit about the fact that everyone's mind is always chattering and generating stories, many of which are very familiar to us and which get replayed over and over. We know that people who struggle with anxiety have a mind that likes to tell scary stories! Often, vivid images accompany those stories.

To illustrate this, I will tell you a story about my own life. Many years ago, when I was training to be a psychologist, I was asked by my clinical supervisor to do a presentation to a group of parents. Although I had some public speaking experience in the past, this was the first time in my clinical training that I was being evaluated on my presentation skills.

As the evening of the presentation drew closer, my anxiety levels started to increase. In the hours before the presentation was due to start, I was experiencing many of the bodily anxiety symptoms that I described in the last chapter. My mind was full of chatter and the main story that was being played out went something like, "You are going to mess this up in front of your supervisor. You are going to get up in front of all those people, and you won't know what to say. They will think that you are an incompetent fool." Coupled with this story was a very vivid image of me standing in front of a group of people stuttering, red-faced, and looking like a fool. Thankfully, despite my nerves, I managed to complete the presentation but the anxiety symptoms were far from pleasant.

We know that when people have difficulties with anxiety, their minds often tell them stories that make their anxiety worse. Just like my experience, these stories and images just add to people's worries, and can be so familiar that we don't even notice them. This is how mindfulness meditation can be helpful; regular practice can help us tune into and notice our thoughts and stories. If we can recognise these stories as *just stories,* we can develop the capacity to prevent ourselves from getting hooked into them and believing them.

In the example from my own life, above, what do you think would have happened if I had really, truly immersed myself in the story that I would mess up the presentation and make a fool of myself? It's likely that I would have made up some excuse to get out of doing it. I would have pretended that I was sick or that there was an emergency at home. This would have been problematic for me in the longer term, as presenting information is a big part of a psychologist's job. Because I knew something about managing anxiety as a result of my training, I recognised that these stories were just stories, generated by my mind in an attempt to keep me safe, to stop me from doing something outside my comfort zone. I knew that my mind, like all minds, was exaggerating the danger.

While this knowledge didn't make the anxiety go away (I was shaking like a leaf when I got up to speak), it did allow me to 'feel the fear and do it anyway'. Because I had developed the capacity to take a step back from my thoughts, to recognise them as just thoughts, my anxiety was unpleasant but I did not avoid what was making me anxious. Incidentally, presenting to groups of people is now a big part of my job and it is one of my favourite things to do at work – this teaches us that…

Anxiety decreases bit by bit if we continue to do what scares us.

Ways to Manage our Tricky Mind

Your mind uses lots of tricks to try to keep you safe.

- Your mind will *exaggerate the danger*. "You will make a fool of yourself," "Everything will go wrong; it always does."

- Your mind will *jump to conclusions*. "That pain in your chest means that you are having a heart attack," "This dizzy feeling means that you are going to faint," "The last time you went for a walk, you paid the price with your pain; if you go for a walk again, you will be crippled for days."

- Your mind thinks that it can *mind read*. "Your boss thinks you are stupid, he regrets hiring you," "People think you are boring."

- Your mind likes to tell you *"what if"* stories, like "What if you have a panic attack in the supermarket?" "What if you go to the party and have to leave early because you are so sore?"

- Your mind likes to *label* you. "You are a born worrier; you always were a worrier and always will be a worrier," "You are such a loser; you could never accomplish that, you are too anxious," "You are not a well man, you couldn't do that."

These anxiety-provoking thoughts fuel the vicious cycle of anxiety. But *we don't have to let this happen*. We can learn to notice the thoughts and recognise them as being thoughts that our mind is generating in an attempt to protect us. We can then have the freedom to decide if we want to take on board the thought, or if we want to just notice the thought but not act on it.

It can also be helpful to consider the costs and benefits to you when you notice an anxiety-provoking story.

In the example from my life, described above, I recognised that if I chose to take on board my anxiety-provoking story ("You are going to mess up"), it could have implications for my career.

Engage in Problem-Solving

We all have things in our life that we worry about from time to time. Some of the things are outside our control, whilst we can potentially change or make others better in some way.

It can be hard to accept that there are some things in life that we cannot change or control. As humans, we don't like uncertainty and things being out of our control; we are much more comfortable dealing with predictable situations. Unfortunately, in a lot of circumstances, we can't have 100% certainty and control, and we cause ourselves *unnecessary* distress trying to achieve it.

However, there are situations in life that cause us to feel stressed or anxious that we *can* do something about.

> **Sometimes there are practical things we can do to help our situation and reduce our worry.**

In this case, adopting a problem-solving approach can be helpful. I have outlined the steps involved in problem-solving below.

1. Identify the problem.

2. Try to list every way that you can think of to overcome the problem. Write down *anything* and *everything*. You might find it beneficial to ask other people for advice.

3. Consider how you have solved similar problems in the past, what your friends and family might advise, and how you would like to see yourself dealing with the problem.

4. Work out the pros and cons of every solution.

5. Pick the solution(s) that works best for you.

6. Break down the solution into smaller, more manageable steps if possible. Move through the steps at your own pace.

Have a Designated Worry Time

Some people find it helpful to have a designated worry time. To do this, you set a convenient time every day to sit down and notice your worries. Fifteen to twenty minutes a day can be set aside for this activity.

You write down your worries and decide if there are any practical solutions to your worries by engaging in some problem solving as described above. Throughout the rest of the day, when you notice that you are worrying, you can silently say to your mind "not now" and come back to the worry at a later time, during your designated worry time.

People who use this technique often report that when they come back to their worries during their designated worry time, they find their concerns from earlier don't seem so important.

If you decide to use this technique, *set a timer* so that your worry time doesn't run over. It is also important to remember that you don't need to use all of your designated worry time. If there are unresolved worries at the end of your worry time, you can 'park' them until the next worry time. You can tell your mind that you will come back to them.

Like most of the techniques outlined in this book, worry time takes practice. When you are experiencing difficulties with anxiety, your mind gets used to generating worrying thoughts, and they just pop into your mind automatically. It can take a while for you to get used to telling your mind to park the worries until your worry time, but like all techniques, it *will* get easier with practice.

Breathe

Look again at the physical symptoms of anxiety. You will see that when you feel anxious, your breathing changes, and your breathing becomes fast and shallow in an attempt to help you fight or flight the danger that your brain perceives. If you can learn to breathe in a different way when you are feeling anxious, it will help you to relax and counteract the anxiety.

Box Breathing

Box breathing can be really helpful when you are feeling anxious. The beauty of this technique is that you can use it anywhere and nobody will know it. You could be standing in a shop queue, waiting at a bus stop, or sitting in the doctor's waiting room when you use it, and the people beside you will not even be aware of it.

It can be helpful to look for a square or rectangular shape in your environment to help you practise this. Look for a door, window, or brick and use that to focus on. Let's use a door as an example. All you do is breathe in as you move your attention up one side of the door, pause or hold your breath as you move your attention across the top of the door, exhale as you move your attention down the other side of the door, and pause or hold your breath as you move your attention across the bottom of the door.

Don't worry too much about the pace of your breathing; as long as it is a little slower and deeper it will be helpful.

If you can't (or don't want to) use a square or rectangle as your focus, you can simply use counting to help you. You could breathe in for the count of three (in: 1, 2, 3), pause or hold your breath for the count of two (hold: 1, 2), exhale for the count of three (out: 1, 2, 3) and pause or hold again for the count of two (hold: 1, 2).

4-7-8 Breathing

This breathing technique can take a little practice. In this exercise, breathing out will take longer than breathing in. This helps your nervous system calm down.

Start by exhaling completely through your mouth, making a whoosh sound. Then close your mouth and inhale quietly through your nose to a mental count of *four*. Next, hold your breath for a count of *seven*. Finally, exhale completely through your mouth, making a whoosh sound to a count of *eight*. This is one cycle. Repeat this cycle for as long as you want.

Sometimes people initially find it hard to do the 4-7-8 exercise, often struggling to exhale for the count of eight. Don't worry if this is the case for you.

You can work your way up to it by doing 3-4-5 breathing. Inhale for the count of *three*, hold for the count of *four*, and exhale for the count of *five*. After you have practised 3-4-5 breathing for a while, try 4-7-8 breathing. Alternatively, just continue practising the 3-4-5 technique.

The Abdominal Lift

You start this exercise standing up. Take four or five deep breaths in preparation for the exercise. Then take another deep breath, blowing all your air out. Imagine that your lungs are balloons where you are emptying all the air. Then hold your breath. As you are holding your breath, suck your belly in and try to focus, particularly on the area below your navel. Hold this position and your breath for a few seconds or as long as you can. Then relax the belly – do this before taking a breath. This is one round of abdominal breathing. Repeat three to five times.

Practise Progressive Muscular Relaxation

Unlike the breathing exercises above, this relaxation exercise is harder to practise when you are "on the go" but it is an exercise that people find useful when they are at home or in a place where they will be undisturbed for a few minutes.

When you are anxious, and when you are in pain, you tense your muscles. It is a normal action, but sometimes people are not even aware of how tense their muscles are.

I can recall an incident from my life that illustrates this. I was travelling home from work several years ago. It was snowing heavily and very quickly the roads became dangerous and slippery. I drove slowly and was very unsure if I should continue driving or just try to pull off the motorway. A journey that normally takes thirty minutes ended up taking four hours. The next morning, when I got up, I had pain in my shoulders and it was sore to move my neck. This pain persisted for a couple of days until it resolved. I realised that for the entire journey home in the snow, my shoulders were up around my ears as I held onto the steering wheel for dear life. I was amazed that this anxiety and muscle tension could have caused such significant pain.

We know that when we are anxious, we tense our muscles. However, we also do this when we *anticipate* a painful experience. If certain movements are painful for you, your muscles likely become tense in anticipation of carrying out that movement. Your brain is once again trying to protect you.

The following exercise can allow us to notice the difference between how muscles feel when they are tense and how they feel when they are relaxed. Every step in this exercise may not be suitable for everyone who has pain, but you can try it and see how you get on. If you find any of the steps aggravate your pain, you can leave them out.

Find somewhere comfortable where you won't be interrupted. Get yourself into a comfortable position; it doesn't matter if you are lying down or sitting. Initially, focus on your breathing; try and slow it down for a few breaths. You could use one of the breathing techniques described above if it helps.

We are going to move through the various muscle groups (listed below). To do this exercise, move through the muscle groups tensing them for about five seconds; you don't have to tense them too tight. Just focus on the sensations in that part of your body. Then, relax your muscles for about five seconds. Again, focus on this part of your body and notice how it feels now. After you have completed this for the first muscle group, move onto the next one. Keep a nice regular breathing pattern going as you move through the muscle groups.

Try not to get too caught up doing it 'right'; just give it a go and see what happens.

You may find it helpful to ask a family or friend to read the instructions below, reminding them that they need to allow about five seconds for each muscle tensing step, and five seconds to notice the relaxation. Alternatively, if you have a smartphone, you could record yourself reading the script onto your phone and then you can play it whenever you want to.

Bring your attention to your face. Make a frowning expression so the muscles in your forehead are tense. Hold for five seconds. Relax. Notice the sensation of relaxation. Squeeze your eyes shut tightly. Hold for five seconds. Relax.

Now move your attention to your jaw. Clench your teeth together. Hold for five seconds. Relax, notice how that feels.

Bring your awareness to your neck. Press your neck back and roll it from side to side slowly and gently. Hold for five seconds, noticing the feeling of tension. Return your neck to its normal position and relax.

Next bring your attention to your shoulders. Lift your shoulders up to your ears. Hold for five seconds. Feel that tension. Drop your shoulders and relax.

Bring your awareness to your chest. Take a deep breath. Hold it for five seconds. Relax and let your breathing return to normal.

Now move your attention to your stomach. Tense your stomach muscles. Hold that tension for five seconds. Relax. Notice the feelings of relaxation.

Move your awareness to your buttocks. Squeeze your buttocks together. Hold for five seconds. Feel that tension. Relax.

Now rest your attention on your legs. Straighten your legs and bend your feet towards your face. Hold for five seconds. Relax. Notice the difference between your feelings of tension and relaxation. Point your toes towards the ground and feel the tension in the back of your legs. Hold for five seconds. Relax.

Move your awareness to your arms. Bend your elbows and move your hands up to your shoulders as if you are lifting a weight. Hold for five seconds, noticing the feelings of tension. Relax.

Finally, switch your focus to your hands. Clench your hands into fists. Hold for five seconds. Relax.

When you have finished this exercise, it can be helpful to spend a few minutes just lying or sitting quietly in a relaxed state. If you notice any more tension in your body, you could try to gently breathe into it, directing your attention into the part of your body where you feel that tension. Alternatively, you can just notice the tension and let it be.

Make Time for Relaxation

When we are stressed or anxious, our bodies release hormones. Cortisol is one of the main stress-response hormones, and has been shown to surge when we are stressed. We are, of course, designed to experience stress in short bursts. Think back to the discussion on the fight or flight response in the previous chapter, where stress helped us escape from or overcome sudden (typically short-lived) danger in the wild.

In modern times, we are constantly encountering stressful situations, and it is possible that we are constantly in flight or fight mode. One of the main ways we have of managing this is to make time for relaxation.

I often ask people what they do for relaxation and fun, and at times, I am met with a blank look. People who live with pain often feel that the fun has gone out of their lives. This may be because they can no longer do the things that they used to enjoy because of their pain. This is especially true if they used sport or physical activity to relax before they developed their pain. If their working life has been impacted by their pain, they may also have had to adjust to a reduced income which can impact the things they do for fun.

Some people believe that it is selfish to prioritise time for relaxation. As a psychologist, I believe that it is not selfish but *essential* to prioritise relaxation in your life. I notice that parents, in particular, seem to struggle with making time for relaxation. It is almost as if they feel every spare minute must be given to their children. When I am discussing this with people, I always use the old metaphor of the air steward on the plane who tells you what to do if you are travelling with children when the oxygen levels in the cabin reduce suddenly. If this happens, we are advised to put on our masks first and then apply the masks to our children. If we don't do this, our life and the lives of our children are at risk. I think that we can use this metaphor to understand how important it is to meet our own needs. If we are unable to put our mask on first (meet our own self-care needs), we are unlikely to be able to meet the needs of the people in our care.

Relaxation is necessary for everyone, irrespective of whether they are living with pain or not. Everyone should make time to relax by doing something enjoyable. It is also important that relaxation is not part of your day 'when you have time'. It should be part of your day, every day. This can help to reduce your anxiety levels by calming the body and mind. It can also help you to sleep. Without taking the time to relax and unwind, it is easy to feel overwhelmed and anxious.

Relaxing activities are very individual. For example, some people find baking relaxing; I just find it stressful, and if you tasted my baking, you would know why! It can be worth trying to develop new activities or try new things to see if you enjoy them, particularly if you had to give up the hobbies that you enjoyed before you developed your pain. I have listed some activities that people have found relaxing, below:

- Reading a book
- Reading a magazine
- Watching a series or box set on TV
- Having a bath
- Cardmaking, knitting, or another creative activity
- Cycling
- Walking
- Yoga
- Woodturning
- Baking
- Cooking
- Painting
- Going to the cinema

- Going for a coffee with a friend

- Gardening

- Playing a musical instrument

- Listening to music

- Colouring in

- Doing a crossword puzzle or sudoku

- Having a massage

Take a moment to list all of the activities that *you* find relaxing. Reflect on how often you incorporate them into your life. If your list isn't very long, take some time to think about whether you could try out any other relaxing activities. Try to prioritise a relaxing activity every day.

Ground Yourself

You will recall that in the chapter on mindfulness that we acknowledged how little time we spend in the present. Often, our minds are focused on the future or are stuck in the past. While we must think about the future and the past, we know that spending a lot of time in the future or past can be very anxiety-provoking. As we discussed, when we are anxious, we can get very caught up in the stories that our minds generate.

Several techniques can be useful when you find your mind is racing with anxiety-provoking thoughts. They will help ground you back in the present.

Focus on your Breathing

For the duration of three breaths (or more if you would like), just focus on your breath. Become aware of the inhale, the pause, and the exhale. It may be helpful to notice where you feel your inhale the most (it may be your stomach, chest, mouth, throat, nose) and where you feel your exhale the most. Unlike the exercises described above, you are *not* trying to change your breathing in any way; you are just noticing the breath. You are bringing your awareness to it.

3-2-1 Noticing Exercise

3-2-1 noticing is another helpful grounding exercise that I described in Chapter 6. Start by noticing three things that you can see, hear, and feel, then notice two things that you can see, hear, and feel, and finally notice one thing that you can see, hear, and feel.

The 3-2-1 noticing exercise will allow your mind to notice what is going on in the present, instead of focusing on the mental drama that your mind is playing out. This exercise will give you a break from the anxiety-provoking story in your mind.

Tackle your Avoidance

As I have mentioned several times, we tend to avoid the things that make us anxious. A trait that is useful in the short-term.

> **However, we know that in the long-term, avoidance makes anxiety worse.**

If you are avoiding important events or activities due to anxiety, you can put a plan in place to manage this avoidance. In the first instance, you should not give yourself a hard time about your avoidance.

> **Remember that avoidance is a normal response to anxiety-provoking situations.**

When psychologists work with people to overcome avoidance, they often ask the person to develop a hierarchy of feared situations and help them work their way through it. To explain this, we can use Jessica as an example.

Jessica and the Step-by-Step Approach to Overcoming Avoidance

Jessica developed difficulties with anxiety after she developed her back pain and sciatica. She had to take a period of extended sick leave from work, and after a few months of not working, she noticed that she became more and more anxious when she was out of the house. Jessica had always been shy and she hated being asked about her pain when she was meeting friends and family. She knew that she still looked well and she worried that people thought that she was exaggerating her pain or that she was looking for attention. She hated the fact that she couldn't walk as fast as her friends and that she sometimes had to go home early on an evening out because she was sore. Over time, Jessica started to avoid social situations, like going shopping and going out for dinner with her family and friends.

Jessica was motivated to work on her anxiety because she was aware that her anxiety was making her pain harder to cope with. She was also aware that her quality of life was diminishing as a result of her pain and anxiety. It was important to Jessica to regularly connect with friends and family, and she knew that her anxiety was preventing her from moving towards this important value.

Jessica listed the situations that were most anxiety-provoking to her. At the bottom of the hierarchy, she had 'meeting my closest friend in my local coffee shop'. This task would be a little difficult for her to manage, but she knew that with effort, she could achieve it. At the top of the hierarchy, she had put her most difficult task, 'going to my cousin's wedding'. When she started her avoidance work, this task seemed nearly impossible to Jessica. Even talking about it made her feel anxious.

In between these two steps, Jessica had several other steps, each one progressively more difficult and anxiety-provoking for her. As part of her therapy, Jessica worked her way through the list that she had set for herself. Once she felt reasonably comfortable completing the easiest step, she moved onto the next one. Like all therapeutic work, it didn't always go to plan, Jessica found some steps harder to achieve and she had to work on accomplishing some steps for longer than others. While Jessica was working through her list, she used the anxiety management skills that she had learned. She practised her breathing, and she worked with the stories that her mind generated.

Summary of the Steps for Working with Avoidance

1. Make a list of the things that you are avoiding.

2. Give everything on your list a score between 0 and 100 depending on how anxiety-provoking they are, with 0 = no anxiety, and 100 = extreme anxiety.

3. Once you have your list of things you are avoiding, construct a ladder or hierarchy. Rank the list in order of difficulty with the thing that has the lowest score (least anxiety-provoking) at the bottom and the situation that has the highest score and is most anxiety-provoking at the top.

4. Start by confronting the lowest-ranked item on your ladder. This is the item that causes you the least anxiety. Keep on this step of the ladder by repeating this step until your anxiety level has reduced by at least half.

   Please remember to be patient and compassionate with yourself as you do this. So often, people have told me that their minds tend to tell very critical stories as they work through their avoidance. If this is the case for you, just notice the stories and acknowledge them for what they are – just old stories being replayed in your mind.

5. If an item on your list seems too difficult, you may have to put in an extra step or two before it. Don't worry about doing this; it is something that people often have to do.

6. Practise working on your avoidance as often as possible. Try to keep the momentum going by repeating the task as often as possible. You will find that your anxiety will gradually decrease over time and your confidence will grow.

7. Remember, as you work through your ladder, to use the anxiety management skills and information that we have discussed in this chapter.

Also, remember that you don't have to fear the symptoms of anxiety; they are just signs that your brain is trying to look out for you. Practise your breathing. Continue to be aware of the thoughts and stories generated by your mind, and remember that you don't have to believe all the stories and rumours that your mind generates..

Consider Reducing your Screen Time

This may not seem relevant, *but it is*, and unsurprisingly it is a technique that most people struggle with.

When I was completing my doctorate training, we had a module on computers. One of the tasks we were given was to find the homepage of the university where I was studying. I wasn't sure how to do this, and I had to ask my classmate who was sitting beside me to help me. I bet you are wondering what century I was born in. It is hard to believe that this was a part of my training at the end of the 1990s. It is amazing how rapidly the internet has grown, and it is unbelievable how much information is now available to us at the touch of a button.

Very few people could now imagine a life without their phone, which is essentially a mini-computer. While there are numerous positives associated with the growth of mobile computing devices – whether phones, tablets or laptops – there are some downsides too. It seems like we are no longer able to rest and be still. In a quiet moment, it is hard not to reach for entertainment and the distraction of a screen. I know that when I am standing in a queue in a shop waiting to pay for something, I have to fight the desire to take out my phone and scroll through Instagram or Facebook. Many people go straight onto their phone or other devices first thing in the morning, often before they have got washed or had breakfast.

In a lot of work environments, it has become expected that you will be available by email well outside your working hours. I believe that this frequent stimulation and lack of time spent in stillness is contributing to our difficulties with anxiety. Our minds are constantly being stimulated; we are not being given the chance to relax properly. We are constantly speeding through our lives.

Humans are designed to have quiet, still time. My grandparents spent their evenings sitting beside the fire, chatting with family or friends who had called to visit. They weren't sitting with their iPads on their knees, scrolling through their social media with one eye and watching the TV with the other eye.

As well as the stimulation provided by mobile devices, I also think it worth considering the impact of social media on our anxiety levels. In the next chapter, I talk about how comparison can contribute to low mood. When we use social media, we will inevitably compare ourselves to others; she has a nicer kitchen than me, he is away on holiday for the third time this year and I can't even afford a week in the sun, she is getting married and I haven't even got a boyfriend, and so on. As well as impacting on our mood, this constant comparison can cause us to feel anxious.

If you want to consider reducing the time that you spend on your electronic device, you could start by reducing the number of notifications that you receive. It can be very hard to ignore the ping of a new notification, but if you turn off your notifications, you will not be prompted to check your phone multiple times per hour. That way, you can begin to control when you want to use your phone.

Many of us sign up to *this* site or *that* newsletter and – before we know it – we get hundreds of emails or messages a day. While I often delete many without reading them, I am conscious that this takes time and effort. It can be helpful to spend some time going through your emails to unsubscribe from those that you no longer want to receive. This can cut down on the information overload that you are faced with every day. It might also be useful to change your email settings so that your emails don't refresh automatically. You can then control *when* you want to check your emails instead of constantly being interrupted by the sound of an incoming email.

It is also worth making meal times electronic-free zones. In the chapter on mindfulness, I mentioned that the practice of mindful eating is now being used to help people with weight management. If we are on our phone when we are eating, we are not eating mindfully; we are not fully aware of what we are eating, nor fully appreciative of the taste and smell of the food as our mind is distracted by our phones.

Ironically, it can be anxiety-provoking to think about withdrawing a little from our phones. As I mentioned a moment ago, it now seems to have become commonplace that people are expected to answer emails almost immediately, whether they are at work or not at work. It can be hard to put down boundaries around this, but if you continue to be available by email, text, or phone almost 24/7, nothing will change and you will never feel like you have any real downtime. I urge you to be protective of your mental health and to consider setting boundaries about your availability. Making a habit of not answering work emails after a certain hour, or on days off, is a good start. Eventually, people will come to accept your new rules regarding your availability.

Change your Posture

Think about the posture of someone who is an anxious state. Imagine you had to go on stage and act like someone who is feeling anxious. What would they look like? I bet you know how easy it is to stand like an anxious person. Have you ever noticed that you may be adopting such a posture yourself, when you are not feeling your best? Be aware of your posture!

There is some evidence to suggest that posture and movement might be able to create emotional states and that they may also be able to reinforce emotional states too.[10] In other words, if you stand like an anxious person, it can make you feel anxious! There is also some evidence that your posture could also change pain sensitivity.[11]

---

[10] Carney, D.R., Cuddy, A. J., Yap, A. J. (2010) Power posing: brief nonverbal displays affect neuroendocrine levels and risk tolerance. *Psychological Science*, 21 (10), 1363-1368.

[11] Bohns, V, Wiltermuth, S. (2012) It hurts when I do this (or you do that): Posture and pain tolerance. *Journal of Experimental Social Psychology*, 48 (1), 341-345.

The next time you are feeling anxious or low in mood, it is worth trying to change your posture. Stand up straight and adopt a confident posture. Imagine that you are on stage and have been instructed to act as if you are oozing confidence. There is some evidence that this posture may also help with pain management. It is something simple and easy to try that may be of some benefit in terms of anxiety, mood, and pain management. Fake it 'til you make it!

Do a Physical Activity

Exercise helps manage anxiety. Nonetheless, I appreciate that when you live with persistent pain, the picture can be a little more complicated than it is for people who don't experience pain. As I outlined in Chapter 4, when you live with pain, even the thought of becoming more active can increase anxiety levels and worry about making the pain worse. However, the research evidence suggests that it is very worthwhile to work on increasing your activity levels. You should try to incorporate regular activity or exercise into your life, even if you are living with pain.

We know that activity and exercise can help reduce muscle tension throughout the body. We also know that exercise produces endorphins. Endorphins are produced within the brain, and the nervous system, and they have several functions. They activate the body's opiate receptors, thereby reducing the perception of pain. They also help in the management of stress and anxiety. Endorphins produce a positive feeling in the body that can explain why seemingly sane people decide to get up at 6 am in the winter to go for a run, and why people spend their weekends hiking mountains or cycling in the rain. Finally, it has been shown that exercise can also decrease the intensity and frequency of panic attacks. So, simply put, exercise can help in the management of pain and anxiety, which is a win-win situation for someone living with pain.

Practise Mindfulness

Yes, I am going to mention mindfulness again! There is a reason that mindfulness appears to be mentioned everywhere these days. As outlined in the mindfulness chapter, mindfulness and the practice of mindfulness meditation has multiple benefits; one of which is its role in the management of anxiety.

Anxiety feels awful, but what is worse, anxiety also changes the structure of our brains. Everyone's brain can change, in good and bad ways, and (as I have explained earlier in this book) this capacity to change is known as neuroplasticity. Anxiety increases the size of your amygdala, the area of your brain responsible for the fear response. This change can lead you to become even more anxious. The good news is that the practice of regular mindfulness meditation has been shown to change the structure of your brain in a positive way and it has also been shown that regular mindfulness meditation reduces levels of the stress hormone cortisol.

Watch your Caffeine Intake

For many people, myself included, caffeine is one of life's pleasures. However, if you are experiencing difficulties with anxiety and pain, you may benefit from reducing your caffeine intake. Drinking too much caffeine can make you more anxious than normal. This is because caffeine can disrupt your sleep and also speed up your heartbeat. (I will talk in more depth about caffeine in the chapter on sleep, but it worth mentioning caffeine here too.) Many people who live with pain become quite reliant on caffeine drinks to give them a lift, especially if sleep is a problem for them.

Avoiding drinks containing caffeine – such as coffee, tea, fizzy drinks and energy drinks – may help to reduce your anxiety levels.

Watch your Alcohol Use

Alcohol is used by millions of people to help them relax and feel more at ease. If you have a social event to go to, it can help you feel more confident. If you are feeling anxious while at home, it can help calm you down and relax. However, we know that these effects are temporary, and over time – if this is your primary way of managing your stress or anxiety – you may find that you are relying on it more and more.

If you are feeling anxious or stressed, keep an eye on your alcohol use. If your alcohol use is increasing as your anxiety gets worse, you could try and implement some of the anxiety management techniques described in this chapter. If you have some different anxiety management tools, you may not need to use alcohol to relax as frequently.

If you think that you are developing a dependence on alcohol, you can get support from your doctor or community organisations.

Coping with Panic Attacks

Some of the readers of this book will experience panic attacks; some will experience them occasionally, while others will experience frequent panic attacks. All of the anxiety management techniques described in this chapter will help you reduce your levels of stress and anxiety. If you experience panic attacks, the techniques described will also assist in reducing the frequency of your panic attacks over time.

In addition to the techniques described above, you could consider using the following techniques when having a panic attack.

- Breathe slowly in through your nose to the count of five. Without pausing, breathe slowly out to the count of five. Continue doing this breathing technique for three to five minutes or for as long as you like.

- Use the grounding technique of noticing things that you can hear, see, and feel.

Many people feel exhausted after a panic attack. When you consider that your body has been in 'fight or flight mode', it is not surprising that you are tired and feel like you have done ten rounds with a sabre-toothed tiger! Try and show yourself some compassion and self-care after a panic attack. It can be worth talking to a friend or family member about your panic attacks so that they can provide you with some support. If panic attacks are becoming a problem in your life, you should seek help from your doctor. They will be able to refer you for professional support.

Seek Professional Support if Needed

You may find that the techniques described in this chapter are enough to help you manage your anxiety. However, you may need more support. In the first instance, you should speak with your family doctor, practice nurse, or other health care provider. You may be referred for individual support with a mental health professional. Most areas have anxiety management groups running, and these can be helpful too.

Please do not suffer in silence. Seek help if you feel you need it. Remember, anxiety and stress make persistent pain much harder to manage, so it is worth developing your anxiety and stress management skills.

Things to Remember

- We can learn how to work with our thoughts and reduce our anxiety.

- Breathing exercises help your body relax and counteract anxiety and stress. It is worth trying a few different breathing exercises to see if there are any that you find particularly helpful.

- Making time for relaxation is *essential* for your well-being.

- Avoidance of anxiety-provoking situations can be overcome with time and determination. Tuning into your values can help you find the motivation to do this.

CHAPTER 9: LOW MOOD AND DEPRESSION

> *Mental pain is less dramatic than physical pain, but it is more common and harder to bear. The frequent attempt to conceal mental pain increases the burden.*
>
> ## C. S. Lewis

A book on pain management would not be complete without a chapter on mood management. Most of my patients have told me that their pain has a negative impact on their mood. I think that anyone who has lived with pain can understand this.

You may not be depressed, and if your mood is generally good, I still think it is important to read this chapter. It contains information that you will find helpful in maintaining good mental health.

Depression is a condition that affects millions of people. It is one of the most common mental health problems worldwide, and the number of people experiencing depression is increasing. According to statistics released by the World Health Organisation in 2020, more than 264 million people of all ages suffer from depression.

Among people who live with persistent pain, depression is even more prevalent than it is among the general population. It is estimated that between 40% and 60% of people who live with persistent pain are depressed.[12]

As I said in a previous chapter, I think it helps to consider mental health as a continuum. It is like a sliding scale, with a notch that moves up or down, indicating how good or poor your mental health is at the time. At times in your life, your mental health will be better or worse; you will move up and down the sliding scale... the 'continuum of mental health'. If you can develop a toolbox of

---

[12] Bair, M. J., Robinson, R. L., Katon, W & Kroenke, K (2003) Depression and comorbidity: A literature review. *Archives of Internal Medicine*, 163, 2433-45.

resources that you can use to move towards better mental health, it will benefit you – whether you are depressed or not.

What is Depression?

Depression is a mood disorder characterised by persistent feelings of sadness, a lack of motivation, and a lack of interest in things. The symptoms of depression range from mild to severe. At its mildest, you may just feel persistently low in mood. At the extreme end of the spectrum, you may feel that you just cannot go on and that life is no longer worth living. When you are depressed, the symptoms can persist for weeks or months and can be so bad that they interfere with your work, family, and social life.

The symptoms of depression can be complex and vary a lot between people. I have listed the symptoms of depression below. Even if you are severely depressed, you may not experience all of them. However, the more symptoms that you have, the more likely it is that you are depressed. If you experience a number of these symptoms for most of the day, every day, for more than two weeks, it is worth seeing your GP or doctor about them if you have not already done so.

Emotions

- Feeling sad or low in mood.
- Feeling guilty.
- Feeling upset, numb, or despairing.
- Losing interest or enjoyment in things.
- Crying a lot or being unable to cry when a sad event occurs.
- Feeling alone even when in company.
- Feeling angry and irritable at the slightest thing.
- Feeling anxious or worried.
- Having low self-esteem.

Physical

- Tiredness.

- Lack of energy.

- Restlessness.

- Sleep problems – finding it difficult to get over to sleep and/or waking up very early in the morning.

- Feeling worse at a particular time of the day; for example, in the mornings.

- Changes in appetite leading to weight gain or loss.

- Poor memory or concentration.

- Aches and pains (even among people who don't live with persistent pain).

- Constipation.

- Reduced interest in sex (low libido).

- Changes to your menstrual cycle.

Behaviour

- Having difficulty making decisions.

- Lacking the motivation to do things, including everyday tasks.

- Putting things off.

- Not doing things that you used to enjoy.

- Withdrawing or cutting yourself off from other people and taking part in fewer social activities.

- Poorer performance at work.

Thoughts

- Losing confidence in yourself.

- Expecting the worst to happen.

- Thinking that everything seems hopeless.

- Thinking that you are helpless.

- Thinking that you hate yourself.

- Thoughts of suicide.

Depression can often come on gradually, so it can be difficult to notice something is wrong. Many people try to cope with their symptoms without realising they are depressed. I have met many people who have been struggling with depression but who had not realised that they *were depressed*. Sometimes, it can take a friend, family member, or professional to suggest something is wrong.

Let's look at the physical symptoms of depression that are listed above. You will see that many of them are also symptoms of persistent pain (like sleep difficulties) and that some of them are also side effects of pain medication (for example, constipation, tiredness, changes in appetite). As a result, it can be difficult for people living with persistent pain – and for the health care professionals working with them – to recognise that the person is suffering from depression.

Causes of Depression

There is no single cause for depression. It can occur for a large number of reasons, and it has many different triggers depending on a person's circumstances. I will discuss some of the factors that can contribute to depression below.

Multiple Stressors

In a previous chapter, I talked about the impact of stressors on our mental health. I explained that if we encounter multiple stressors, we may go on to develop difficulties with anxiety and depression. Common stressful life events – like separation, divorce or bereavement – can contribute to the development of depression.

Living with persistent pain is undoubtedly a significant stressor and you can develop difficulties with depression and/or anxiety as a result. For example, let us consider the experience of a person we will call Max.

When Max developed persistent pain, he began to withdraw from friends, conserving all his energy for work. He was unable to engage in his hobby of playing indoor football two evenings a week, due to his pain, and he began to drink more in an attempt to manage his pain and improve his sleep, which had deteriorated since he developed his pain. This led to a 'downward spiral' of events that eventually led to Max becoming depressed.

Adverse Childhood Experiences

A lot of research has been carried out on the impact of adverse childhood events or ACEs on a person's wellbeing in later life. ACEs are potentially traumatic events that occur in a child or adolescent's life before they are aged 18. Physical, emotional, and sexual abuse are considered to be ACEs. Experiencing domestic abuse or living with an adult who was a problem drinking is also regarded as an ACE. Parental separation or divorce or feeling that no one in your family loved you or thought that you were important or special is an ACE.

The number of ACEs experienced by someone has a graded relationship to both the prevalence and the severity of depressive symptoms. However, it is important to note that not all children who experience early life stress go on to develop depression or other difficulties with their mental health. Having a significant adult (for example, a grandparent) who loves you, or having a teacher who understands and encourages you, or having a close friend who provides you with emotional support can help mitigate against the effects of these adverse experiences.

Personality

Some people have low self-esteem and tend to be highly critical of themselves. They may be this way because of their experiences when they were growing up. They may have experienced serious adverse events in childhood, like trauma and neglect.

Other people may not have experienced any serious events like this, but they may not have had the emotional support and positive reinforcement from their caregivers that they needed. Decades ago, when many of my patients grew up, parents and teachers were less aware of the importance of praising and encouraging children for achieving small things or for trying hard. Some people's lack of confidence dates back to their childhood, when responsible adults simply didn't do enough to encourage children and build up self-esteem.

When people develop persistent pain, their self-esteem can deteriorate further and they can become even more self-critical.

Low self-esteem and a tendency towards self-criticism can be significant factors that contribute to the development of depression.

Family History

If a close family member has a history of depression, it is more likely that you will also develop difficulties with depression. However, it is important to remember that even if you have a family history of depression, *it is by no means inevitable* that you will develop difficulties with depression yourself.

Illness

People who have had a serious illness or a condition such as coronary heart disease or cancer have a higher risk of developing depression. Other conditions like an underactive thyroid (hypothyroidism) can place you at greater risk of developing depression.

Loneliness

In recent times there has been a lot of discussion in the media about loneliness. The headlines scream about a 'loneliness epidemic' and it appears that more and more of us feel lonely and disconnected from others, no matter how many friends we have on social media. The need for humans to connect with others is innate; we need human connection to maintain good mental and physical health.

We know that people can feel lonely even if they are around other people; for example, someone who is trapped in an unhappy marriage may feel the burden of loneliness. It is possible that someone who has family and friends who are great fun to have a gossip with, can still lack people to share worries or fears with. Loneliness can increase your risk of developing depression.

Alcohol/Drug Use

When life is hard, and when we feel down, we try to do what we can to cope with it. Many people 'drown their sorrows' with alcohol to numb their feelings and try to escape their low mood. Some people use illicit or prescription drugs to try and cope.

Unfortunately, this only provides a short-term fix and we know that drugs and alcohol often make depression worse.

Depression and Persistent Pain

As I mentioned earlier on in this chapter, while depression is common in the general population, it is even more common among people who live with persistent pain. We know that some people become depressed after they develop their pain, while others may have been depressed before they developed their pain.

When I consider the high prevalence of depressive episodes among people living with pain, one of the biggest factors that contribute to the development of depression is the *multiple losses* that people living with persistent pain have to endure. When people first develop their pain, they are often hopeful that their pain will follow the pattern of acute pain; that is, they hope that their pain will improve over weeks or months and that it will eventually resolve. However, as their pain persists, they can begin to experience a large number of losses: loss of self-confidence, loss of social life, loss of hobbies and interests, loss of employment, and financial loss. Their self-concept can change; they no longer feel like the person they were before they developed their pain.

In my experience, people who live with persistent pain can struggle with the changes to their identity. For example, many patients tell me they have struggled with the impact that their pain has had on their working lives, their ability to provide financially for their family, their identity as 'a breadwinner'. Others have told me that they have struggled with the fact that they now need emotional and practical help and support, themselves. This is particularly true for people who, before they developed their pain, regarded themselves as a person that *others could turn to for help*.

Grieving for the loss of something or someone that is valued is a normal human response. Loss and grief can be a fundamental part of living with persistent pain. The picture is complicated by the fact that pain can be a hidden condition. If you endure a 'public' loss – like the death of a partner – that loss and your grieving will be acknowledged by friends, family, and colleagues. When you live with persistent pain, your losses and associated grieving may not even be noticed or fully appreciated by others. This lack of acknowledgement can be particularly difficult to cope with, and can make it even harder to grieve.

People can change how they think about themselves when they live with pain and depression. Thoughts like, "I am useless," "I am a burden," "I am not a good partner," "I am a failure," "I am a disappointment" are common. We know that when we are depressed, we can get very caught up and 'fused' with the stories that our minds generate about how useless or powerless we are. We can fuse with stories about how hopeless our future is, and feel disempowered and helpless. Everything can become a struggle; even getting up, getting showered and dressed can feel like it requires superhuman effort.

Thoughts and Depression

Let's look a little closer at the role that thoughts play in depression and low mood. We know that everyone has negative thoughts. However, we also know that people who are depressed are more troubled by negative thoughts. Often, they pay more attention to their negative thoughts and get caught up in them. People sometimes think that a person who is depressed could, and should, just learn to stop these thoughts in their tracks, to stop them from forming in the first place. Unfortunately, it is not as easy as that.

Psychologists describe such negative thoughts as 'automatic', because they just pop into our minds instinctively. When people are depressed, they can develop unhelpful thinking styles. Earlier in this book, I mentioned an unhelpful thinking style, one that I notice a lot among people who live with pain; that is the tendency to 'mind-read' – to assume that they know what others are thinking about them. I will talk a little more about this, below. There are also a lot of other unhelpful thinking styles that people have.

Comparing Yourself Negatively to Others

It is human nature to compare ourselves to others. We all do it; we are hard-wired to do so. There are some positives associated with comparing ourselves to others. However, when we compare ourselves to others, we often perceive ourselves to be lacking in some way.

> *Comparison is the thief of joy.*
> ## Theodore Roosevelt

You have probably come across this quotation before, but I think it is worth considering. Many times, I hear people comparing themselves to others and concluding that they – or their lives – are lacking in important ways. This can be particularly true for people who are living with depression.

Emma was 18 when she injured her shoulder in a horse riding accident. She had lived with persistent pain in her shoulder since the fall two years ago. Emma had become increasingly aware of the comparisons she made when she used social media. When she went online and checked her social media accounts, everyone seemed to be living 'their best life'. Everyone appeared happy and seemed to be living fulfilled lives. Her life was difficult and stressful in comparison. She noticed that when she compared her life to that of her friends, as portrayed on social media, her mood was lower.

I know that Emma is not alone in noticing this lowering of mood when she uses social media. I think that many people forget that people always show their 'best face' in public and that nobody, no matter how healthy or wealthy they are, lives a charmed life.

Everyone has stressors to cope with in life. That picture of the perfect family holiday doesn't show the reality of a grumpy teenager, a tired toddler, or a hot and hassled mother. It is just a snapshot that is not reflective of reality. This was brought home to me a couple of years ago when I was on holiday. I overheard a conversation between a young woman and someone who I assumed was her partner. She was asking him to take photographs of her so that she could post one on her Instagram account. Eventually, after about fifteen minutes, much posing, a few irritable exchanges – and what appeared to be hundreds of photographs – she seemed satisfied with one photograph. The people viewing that photograph only saw the finished product and not the 'real life' that went on behind it. They only saw a heavily edited view of that one day on holiday.

If you notice that your mood is lower after using social media, consider taking a break from it or not following those people who make you feel less than adequate. Some people have stopped using social media completely, and they report that their mood is better as a result. Consider whether this might be an option for you.

Even if you don't use social media, I am quite sure that you frequently compare yourself to other people. Many patients have spoken to me about the stories that this comparison generates in their minds. "Joanne brought her daughters for a full day shopping. You are an awful mother; all you can manage is a couple of hours in the shops" or "the Jones are going to Florida for a big family holiday. My children are never going to get to do that because I am only able to work part-time because of my pain" or "Rebecca is twenty years older than me, and she is so much fitter," and so on and so on.

By tuning into your mental chatter, you can begin to notice these comparison stories. By becoming more aware of your comparison stories, you can stop yourself from getting hooked on them, and this can help stop you from spiralling into negativity.

Mind Reading

As I stated before, we often engage in mind reading – we assume that we know what other people are thinking. Often, this mind reading is focused on what others are *thinking* about us, and we typically assume that their thoughts about us are negative or critical in some way.

For example, you may notice somebody watching you walk slowly and believe, "They think that I am putting this on, that I am only looking for attention" or "He thinks there is nothing wrong with me, that I am just being lazy."

Psychologists know that people are *very poor* mind readers, that non-verbal communication is hard to interpret, and that we often make mistakes when we try to work out what other people are thinking. My experience is that mind reading can be problematic for people who live with pain; they can start avoiding social contact as they believe that other people are judging them or thinking negatively about them. This avoidance of social contact can have a very significant negative impact on psychological wellbeing and quality of life. As I said earlier in this chapter, social contact and staying in touch with family and friends are very important for a person's wellbeing.

You can work with your tendency to mind read by becoming aware of your thoughts. If you notice that you have started to 'mind read', you can take a break from it by bringing your awareness back to your breath or your body. By becoming aware of your breath – even for the duration of just three breaths – you can break that cycle of negative thinking. By bringing your awareness back to your body, by noticing how your feet feel on the ground, or the contact that your body is making with the chair, you can prevent the escalation of suffering by *stopping* your thoughts and stories taking over.

Mental Filter

You have probably heard the old saying about seeing the world through 'rose-tinted glasses'. We all wear glasses or use a lens when we think about ourselves, the world, and our future. Our beliefs colour the way that we see the world. When someone's mood is low, they are drawn towards noticing the negative aspects of life.

When you are living with pain every day, it is very easy to get drawn into only noticing how difficult life is, and failing to see the more positive aspects of your life.

It can feel as though a negative filter has permanently slid across your mind's eye. When you have your negative mental filter in place, your mind can generate all sorts of stories to explain why positive events don't count; for example, "My friend really didn't enjoy my company tonight, she was just being nice when she said that she had a good time."

It can be helpful to become aware of your thoughts and *notice* when you are using a negative mental filter to look at the world.

Critical Self

As I have said before, most of us have an internal critic – that voice that likes to put us down and criticise. When you become more aware of your thoughts, you develop the capacity to notice self-critical stories. You may notice that you apply labels to yourself, for example, labelling yourself by saying things such as, "I am a total idiot," "I am a waste of space," "I am pathetic."

You may have noticed that since you developed persistent pain, your internal critic has become very vocal; frequently commenting on what you can no longer do and what you *should* be doing. Often this critic will refer back to your life before pain and compare what you are doing now with your previous life. The internal critic does not carry out this comparison in a compassionate and supportive way; it does so in a harsh, judgemental way.

By becoming aware of your thoughts, you will be able to recognise when this internal critic is to the fore. If you develop the capacity to observe the critic, you are less likely to get drawn into the stories he/she tells you, and you will be better able to see the criticism for what it is; stories and projections in your mind.

Catastrophising

If your mood is low, or if you are depressed, you are likely to catastrophise about your situation. We all catastrophise at times, and when we catastrophise, we make things out to be much worse than they really are. For example, you might make a mistake at work and get caught up in stories of how you are going to lose your job as a result. If you are experiencing a flare-up of your pain, you might get caught up in thoughts like, "This is awful, I can't stick another minute of this" and "I can't go on like this" or "What if this never ends, what if the pain doesn't ease?"

Again, developing the capacity to become aware of your thoughts and making the decision to bring your awareness back to your body or your breath, even for a few moments, can prevent you from getting caught up in those stories in your mind. You can learn to become an observer of your mind and, in doing so, begin to recognise that this is the 'catastrophising' passenger in your mind speaking. You can remember that you, like all people, are *wired to overestimate threat* and that you can choose not to take on board your mind's dire predictions.

All or Nothing Thinking

We know that thinking in an 'all or nothing' way can have a negative impact on our mood. We can use Jane's experience as an example of this.

Jane was very close to her cousin. Her cousin's hen party involved an outdoor activity centre for the day, followed by dinner and drinks in the evening with an overnight stay. Jane was very dismayed when she heard about the activities planned for the hen party and decided to cancel, due to her inability to participate in the daytime activity because of the pain she suffered. She immediately discounted the fact that she *could* fully take part in the *rest* of the hen party but – in her mind – if she couldn't take part in all of the hen party, she wasn't taking part in any of it.

When Jane reflected on this, she realised that she was missing out on an important event in her life and that she could *choose* to listen to her inner voice saying, "There is no point in going unless you can take part in it all" or she could *choose* to move towards her values and attend the hen night. In the end, she attended the hen night and was glad to enjoy this special event with her cousin.

In this chapter, we have looked at the symptoms of depression and some of the causes of depression. We have also explored how thoughts influence mood.

In the next chapter, I will explore strategies that have been shown to help manage difficulties with low mood and depression and improve mental health.

Things to Remember

- Depression is one of the most common worldwide mental health problems.

- It is estimated that between 40 and 60% of people who live with persistent pain are depressed.

- Multiple factors lead someone to develop difficulties with depression.

- Everyone experiences negative thoughts. People who are depressed are more troubled by them, and they engage in unhelpful thinking styles more frequently than others who are not depressed.

- If you believe that you are depressed, or experiencing low mood, turn to the next chapter to discover some strategies that have consistently been shown to help manage these difficulties.

CHAPTER 10: MANAGE YOUR MOOD

> *There is hope, even when your brain tells you there isn't.*
>
> ## John Green

As I explained in the previous chapter, when your mood is low, or when you are depressed, things can seem pretty hopeless. It is important to remember that hopelessness is a symptom of depression, and there are many things that you can do to improve your life, even if you are depressed and in pain.

In this chapter, we shall explore strategies that have been shown to help people manage their low moods and depression.

> **Even if you are not depressed, I urge you to read this chapter. It contains information that will help you maintain good mental health.**

Develop a Routine and Make a Daily Plan

When you are in pain, and you are depressed, everything can feel like an effort. Even getting out of bed in the morning and getting washed and dressed can be exhausting. If you look at the symptoms of depression (in the previous chapter), you will see that difficulty motivating yourself is one of them. It can be hard to work up the motivation to do even the simplest thing.

People who are in pain often find that any routine is hard to maintain. For example, if they have had a tough night, and have slept badly, it can be hard to get up at their set time in the morning unless they need to go to work or get children on their way to school. Many patients have told me that their days are unstructured; that one day blurs into the next. This is particularly true for people who are no longer in employment.

Make Plans to Get into a Routine

It is important to try to get yourself back into a routine. To do so, it can be useful to develop a daily and weekly plan. As advocated in Chapter 5, try to spend some time before the start of a new week, or before going to bed at night, planning some activities for the week or day ahead. Your plan could be quite detailed or you could start by planning just a few activities.

Everyone's starting point for their plan will be different. I have worked with many people who were experiencing severe depression. Their first plan might be to get dressed by 11 am two days a week. As they achieve this goal, they begin to plan more and more things for their week.

I have worked with other people who have managed to hold down busy full-time jobs despite their depression and pain. However, they noticed that all they were doing was working and that all the pleasure had gone out of their lives. Their weekly plan involved scheduling some pleasurable, fun activities.

Let's take Holly as an example. Holly might plan something like this: on Monday, Wednesday and Friday I am going for a walk. On Thursday, I am going to meet a friend for coffee. On Saturday evening, I am going to go out for a meal with my partner. I am going to practise ten minutes of mindfulness meditation every day.

As I have said before, it can be particularly difficult for people who live with pain to plan activities as they may experience a flare-up in their pain and be unable to stick with their plan. Often, people completely give up planning activities because of this.

People with pain and depression can still plan and develop routines, but it is important that this planning is done with flexibility. You will remember how I wrote, previously, that psychologists know that developing psychological flexibility is very important, especially for people living with pain. Psychological flexibility means that you learn to adapt to life's curveballs.

Let's go back to that plan above. Imagine that Holly went for her walk on Monday – as planned – and it went well. She felt great afterwards and felt like she had accomplished something. She also managed to complete her walk on Wednesday as planned. However, on Thursday she experienced a flare-up in her pain. Holly struggled to get up and dressed, and she decided to cancel her coffee date with her friend. What might Holly's inner voice have to say in this situation? Perhaps things like, "What was the point in arranging to meet for coffee? You should have known you wouldn't be able to make it," "You are such a chump, your friend Charlotte had arranged for her mother to babysit so she could meet you and then you ended up letting her down. You are a pathetic friend; you can't even meet Charlotte for a coffee."

If Holly really listened to these stories from her inner voice, what would happen to her mood? She would feel even lower! Do you think that she would be more or less likely to go back to her plan when her flare-up settled? In all likelihood, she would be less likely to go back to her plan, probably thinking that planning activities are pointless.

But what if there is another way for Holly? It would be helpful if she didn't listen to the chatter in her mind, and recognise that she does not have to respond to the chatter. Holly could recognise that she is in charge of her life and is 'driving her bus'. She can choose to accept that her inner voice is playing out old, familiar stories that are not helpful. She can choose just to notice those thoughts. Holly could show some self-compassion; she could recognise that she had a bad day and that she did her best on that day. This would make it much more likely that Holly would plan activities again and arrange another coffee date with Charlotte.

Holly's thoughts and self-criticism are very typical of someone living with depression. People can have very powerful beliefs that colour how they view every situation that they encounter in life. You will remember that our minds cannot remember everything that happens to us.

> Like a good film editor, our minds will edit
> the story of our lives to provide a coherent
> story that is consistent with our beliefs.

People who are depressed can have very negative and inflexible beliefs and thoughts about themselves; for example, they might believe "People don't like me," "I am pretty useless at everything," "I let everyone down," "I am a bad mixer," "I should be able to provide for my family," "I should be able to look after my grandchildren." Additionally, they can have negative beliefs and thoughts about the world and the future, "People are so selfish," "Everything goes wrong for me," "Things will never get any better for me."

We know that there is a tendency for people to filter out their experiences that do not fit with these beliefs and to focus on the experiences that seem to confirm what they think about themselves. As such, try to understand that your mind can play tricks on you and steer you towards negative thoughts. Be aware of your negative inner voice, but recognise that it often *exaggerates* the negatives. You can choose to hear what your inner voice says but you don't have to take it on board or really 'listen' to it.

Stay In Touch with Family and Friends

If you have another look at the symptoms of depression, you will see that withdrawal from others is one of its prominent features. This withdrawal can take many forms; for example, many people have told me that they have withdrawn from their partner and family members at home. They might, for example, go into another room or their bedroom to watch TV alone in the evenings while the rest of their family are in the living room together. People can also withdraw from others by not answering phone calls or text messages. They may withdraw from their usual social activities of meeting their friends for coffee, lunch, a game of cards, or a few drinks.

There is an old saying, 'it is good to talk', and we know that social support and staying in touch with people is very important for our mental health. Psychologists recognise that social support is a buffer to mental health problems, but it can sometimes be difficult to reach out to others for support, especially when you are depressed. Simply put, you may feel exhausted and struggle to get the energy to connect and meet up with other people.

Despite the effort involved, it can be helpful to choose at least one person to open up to – to discuss your difficulties with – in a more intimate way. People often tell me that they don't like doing that; their family member or friend has enough to cope with in their day-to-day life, without them being burdened further.

When I hear this, I know that the person I'm speaking with probably has beliefs like, "It is weak to lean on others" or "It is selfish to tell other people about my problems" or that "You should always be strong and manage on your own." It is worth remembering that true intimacy – be it with a partner, family member or friend – is about sharing that vulnerable part of you and also being available as a support to that other person. If you are courageous and open up to someone now, you may free that person up to lean on you for support when they need it. Life throws curve balls at all of us, and while you may need support at present, there is likely to come a time when you will be the person that is providing the support.

> **Giving back to others is very good for our psychological wellbeing.**

Sometimes, people feel that they have lost touch with their friends and family. If you have had your pain for a while, you may be unable to work because of your pain and may have lost touch with former colleagues.

If you feel you have lost touch with your friends, family, or former colleagues, you could think about reconnecting with them. This could initially be done via a text message or social media message as that is often the easiest first step. However, we know that face to face contact is the most beneficial form of contact for people; try to find a way to eventually arrange to meet up in person.

Increase Your Activity Levels

I have already spent quite a bit of time discussing the benefits associated with becoming more active. We know that exercise is beneficial in the management of depression and that *any* increase in activity levels will do you good. You do not need to be sweating it out in the gym or running around the park in skin-tight lycra to profit from becoming more active.

Remember that your mind is likely to tell you stories about how pointless it is to increase your activity levels or how unsafe it is to do so. Remember that these stories are generated by your mind to keep you within your comfort zone.

> **Also, remember that the reason you are reading this book is because you want to move outside your comfort zone and live a better life.**

People often tell me that fatigue is a big problem for them. Whilst fatigue and tiredness are symptoms of depression, fatigue is also associated with persistent pain. When you are living with pain, and when you are also tired and depressed, it can be difficult to start becoming more active. As stated in the chapter on activity, even though it appears counterintuitive, studies indicate that your *fatigue will lessen* the more active you become.

It can be helpful to think about your whole life as a workout. Could you walk a little further to work in the morning? Could you walk around a few more shops in the shopping centre?

When you increase your activity levels, it is vital that you pace your activity, so be sure to read Chapter 5 on pacing and rule-breaking so you can gradually become more confident in your abilities. You do not need to do a day's 'exercise' all in one go. For example, you could do an extra five minutes in the morning, an extra five minutes at lunchtime, and another seven minutes in the afternoon. This adds up to another seventeen minutes of activity.

Physical activity and exercise can often involve social interaction as well. There are a lot of benefits associated with exercising with someone else. For example, if you regularly go for a walk with a friend, you are less inclined to avoid it if your mood is low, and you are struggling to motivate yourself. When you are walking with your friend, there is the opportunity to connect with them and relax and have a chat, both of which improve your mental health.

Become Mindful

Many people find that adding a mindfulness element to their activity is helpful. This can be particularly positive if you find yourself stuck in a cycle of repeatedly thinking about your problems.

To become more mindful of your activity, you can focus on what you are doing in the here and now. For example, if you are going for a walk, you could think about the sensation of your feet hitting the ground, the sensation of the sun on your back, or (if you live in the UK) the sensation of the rain on your face!

You could become more aware of the sounds that you hear, and notice what you can see and even smell. You could become aware of your breathing as you walk – the inhale, the pause, and the exhale. So much of the time, we are stuck in our heads – on autopilot – listening to the incessant chatter of our minds. Our minds are 'full', rather than 'mindful'. Engaging in mindful activity can give us a break from the stories of our mind; it can help the mental chatter fade into the background, at least for a while.

As I explained in the chapter on mindfulness, we don't even need to be engaging in 'exercise-type activity' to practise mindfulness. For example, you could practise mindful awareness when you are in the shower, noticing the sensation of the warm water on your back, the smell of the shampoo as you wash your hair, etc. While this mindful activity is not attempting to get rid of your depression or negative thoughts, it will give your mind a break from ruminating or going over and over stories and negative thoughts in your mind.

Practise Mindfulness Meditation

I have already talked about becoming mindful in this chapter. I am going to mention the benefits of mindfulness meditation again(!) as we know that mindfulness meditation is effective in the management of depression and mood problems.

When you are depressed, it is hard to work up the motivation to do anything – even the essential things in life. Whatsmore, it can be especially difficult to work up the motivation to practise even a few minutes of mindfulness meditation. However, the evidence is clear, and I urge you to consider trying to practise it. Even five to ten minutes a day, a couple of times a week, is a great start.

Many people have told me that it is hard to remember to practise meditation. To help you remember, anchor it to something that you are already doing routinely, like brushing your teeth. If you associate meditation with brushing your teeth in the morning, you are much more likely to remember to do it.

Practise Gratitude

Research suggests that the feeling of gratitude may be associated with many benefits for individuals, including better physical and psychological health and increased happiness and life satisfaction.

In one particular study that was carried out with people who had mental health concerns, it was found that the people who practised gratitude – by writing gratitude letters – had significantly better mental health four weeks and twelve weeks after their writing exercise ended.[13] The authors of this study suggest that 'gratitude letter writing' improves mental health by shifting one's attention away from negative emotions, such as resentment and envy. They believe that when you write about how grateful you are to others, and how much other people have blessed your life, it might become considerably harder for you to ruminate, or

---

[13] Wong, Y. W., Owen J., Gabana, N. T., Brown, J. W., McInnis, S., Toth, P & Gliman, L (2018) Does gratitude writing improve the mental health of psychotherapy clients? Evidence from a randomized controlled trial. *Psychotherapy Research*, 28:2, 192-202.

repeatedly think, about your negative experiences. Since our brains have a natural tendency to focus on threats, worries, and negative aspects of life, feeling and expressing gratitude can help direct our attention to the positive.

> **Negative thoughts can stick like Velcro, while positive thoughts can be like Teflon.**

By focusing on gratitude, you can begin to experience more emotions like joy, love, and contentment. Fostering gratitude can also create a positive cycle of thinking and behaving in healthy, positive ways.

You will probably not notice any benefits from the practice of gratitude overnight. Like most of the tools in this book, it takes perseverance. The good news is that it only takes five to ten minutes a day to practise gratitude, and in as little as two to three weeks of daily practice, you should notice the benefits.

Types of Gratitude Practices

Several gratitude practices are beneficial. Let's run through them now.

Gratitude Diary

Keep a diary of the things that make you feel grateful. Write down three things that you are grateful for every day. For example, if you have a warm bed to sleep in, you could be grateful for that; if you turn on the switch and the light comes on, you could be grateful for that. If you have clothes and shoes to wear, you could be grateful for them. If you have food to eat, you could be grateful for that. You could be grateful for all the people that have helped get the food to your table. This might include the farmers who grew the food, the drivers who transported it, the factory workers who packaged it, and so on.

You could be grateful for the people in your life who provide you with love and support. Alternatively, you could be grateful for your sight or your hearing. It may seem difficult to imagine being able to find three things every day to be grateful for, but you will be surprised how easy it is when you sit back and reflect on your life. As part of this practice, you need to think about *why* you are grateful for that particular thing. Spend a moment feeling the emotion of that gratitude.

At the end of the day, before you go to sleep, you could reflect on your day and be thankful for the best thing that happened that day. Think about the good things in your day and choose one to focus on in particular. Even on the worst of days, there will always be something to be thankful for.

Write a Gratitude Letter

Write a letter to someone who has been a positive influence in your life or who has provided you with love and support. This could be a parent, sibling, partner, friend, former teacher, colleague, or somebody else. Map out *why* you are grateful to them in the letter.

You can send the letter if you wish (but you don't have to send it, and you will still benefit from this practice even if it never leaves your possession).

Arrange a Gratitude Visit

Visit someone that you are grateful for. Tell them why you are grateful for them. If you want, an additional step is to write a gratitude letter and give it to them during the visit.

Get a Daily Dose of Sunshine

When we consider the things that can help to keep our minds and our bodies well, it is worth considering what our hunter-gatherer ancestors did with their time. When they wanted a steak, they did not use their smartphone to order it from the online supermarket! They went outdoors and hunted for it.

Our bodies remain much the same as when our forefathers were hunter-gatherers; this means we are built for some outdoor living. We are not designed to sit in artificially-lit, centrally heated homes all day. Sunlight is good for us.

There is evidence that sunlight can boost serotonin levels and improve your mood. Serotonin is the brain chemical that is most directly linked to mood, and many anti-depressants work by boosting levels of serotonin in the brain. Higher levels of serotonin correspond with better moods and feelings of satisfaction and calmness; lower levels of serotonin are associated with depression and anxiety.

In the part of the world where I live, the sun is rarely present, and I could be forgiven for skipping this piece of advice (indeed, the sky is grey and cloudy for about nine months of the year). However, research indicates that it doesn't matter if it is cloudy or even raining. You need to get outside and embrace the sunlight.

It is good for our brains to be outside.

Light is measured in units called lux. Bright sunlight – typical of a lovely, bright, sunny day – gives us about 30,000 lux. Going outside on a cloudy day provides approximately 10,000 lux. If you are inside, in a brightly lit room, you will be getting about 500 lux. If you spend most of your time indoors, your body's rhythms may well be disrupted. This can have a particularly detrimental impact on your sleep. I have written a separate chapter on sleep, but it is worth mentioning this important benefit of sunlight exposure here as well.

If possible, try and get outside for at least 20 minutes every day without sunglasses. Morning light is particularly advantageous to us, so it can be worth making a real effort to get outside in the morning, even in the winter. Many patients, who can no longer work, tell me that they are rarely outside, especially in the winter. Often, they get up and spend most of the day at home, except when they go to the shops or to see friends or family. People who are able to work – myself included – often leave home, travel by car or train to their workplace and travel home again, without seeing daylight during the winter months. This pattern is common.

You can try and get more natural sunlight in a variety of ways. For example, you could consider having your morning cup of tea or coffee outside. This is easy in the summer but not so enticing in the winter! However, if you focus on the potential benefits to your mental health and sleep, you may find the motivation to wrap up warm and go outside for your morning cuppa.

You could also consider going for a walk outside or spending some time sitting in your garden or on a park bench. You may decide that you can spend 20 minutes a day doing some gardening, thereby getting your sunlight exposure as well as engaging in physical activity and getting some work done.

Keep an Eye on Your Alcohol Intake

When we feel bad, it is normal to want something that takes away the difficult feelings. Alcohol is often used by people to provide some relief when they have had a bad day or when their mood is low. People who are having difficulties sleeping because of pain and depression, sometimes use alcohol to help them sleep. While this can seem like a good solution in the short-term, it can add to people's difficulties, leading people to feel even more depressed.

It can be useful to reflect on your alcohol use. Has your alcohol intake increased over time? Has a glass of wine in the evening become half a bottle or a full bottle? Has a couple of beers at the weekend become beers most evenings?

If you are concerned about how much you are drinking, you could set a goal to reduce your drinking. We discuss goal setting in a later chapter. If you find this too difficult on your own, you can ask your GP or doctor for help, or you can research support organisations in your area.

Take Your Medication as Prescribed

If you are on anti-depressant medication, you should take it as prescribed. If you are feeling better and think that you may want to come off your anti-depressant medication, it is important that you seek medical support. Don't stop taking your anti-depressant medication abruptly. Your doctor will be able to guide you through this process.

Seek Professional Support

If you think that you may be depressed and struggling to cope, you should seek professional support. The support that people require varies, depending on the nature of their difficulties. Your GP or other health care provider should be able to provide you with advice about accessing support in your local area.

As I mentioned at the start of this chapter, people may feel that their life is so hard that there is no point in living. They can think that their emotional and physical pain is unbearable, and it can be difficult for them to imagine it ending. People can feel useless and unneeded by other people, and they can feel desperate and believe that ending their life is the only way out of their suffering.

If you are feeling like this, it is essential to remember that *you deserve support and that there is support available to you.* Talk to friends, a family member, and your doctor about how you are feeling. This can feel like a daunting prospect; many people are worried that others will be angry with them for feeling like this. Other people have told me that they don't want to burden their friends or family member or cause them to worry. However, reaching out for help is the first step to feeling better.

If you don't feel like you can keep yourself safe, it is important to seek help immediately. You can get an emergency appointment from your GP or go to the Emergency Department of your nearest hospital. Some organisations offer support by telephone. In the UK, you can contact the Samaritans 365 days a year, anytime day or night, for free on any phone on 116 123. There is a misconception that you need to be suicidal to call the Samaritans. While they can provide support to someone who is suicidal, they can also offer a listening ear to anybody who is struggling. Many people have told me that they have contacted the Samaritans when they have been having a bad day, and it has been really helpful to get the support of someone who will listen without judgement.

Things to Remember

- When you are depressed, life can appear hopeless. However, there are many strategies that you can use to help manage your depression.

- If your mental health is good, using the strategies discussed in this chapter will help you stay well.

- Living with persistent pain and depression can seem overwhelming at times, but it is important to remember that you can recover from depression and that professional help is available if you need it.

CHAPTER 11: SLEEP BETTER

> *Sleep is the best meditation.*
> **The Dalai Lama**

Gary has significant sleep problems. Before going to bed, he usually watches TV, often scrolling through Facebook at the same time. He frequently dozes off on the sofa, but when he goes to bed, Gary suddenly feels wide awake. He stays in bed, tossing and turning, his mind racing while trying not to wake his wife, who has to get up early for work. He often feels like he watches every hour pass by on the clock, and as the hours tick by, he becomes more and more anxious about his inability to get to sleep.

Pauline is living with persistent shoulder pain. Most of the time, she has no difficulty falling asleep, but she often wakes in pain during the night. Sometimes, she struggles to get back to sleep.

I would guess that everyone reading this book has had nights of sleeplessness like Gary and Pauline. I know that I certainly have. Sleep, or lack of adequate sleep, is a difficulty experienced by most people at some time in their lives. It is even more common among people who live with persistent pain. No book on pain management would be complete without a chapter on sleep.

We are now sleeping less than ever before. For example, in the 1940s, adults got – on average – 7.9 hours of sleep a night. Today, the average adult in the UK receives 6.5 hours sleep.

There are several reasons why we are sleeping less than before. Many people are working longer hours than ever. In a previous chapter, I mentioned the culture of being available by email, text, or phone 24/7. Many of us check our phone and emails last thing before we go to sleep and first thing in the morning, often before we have even had a shower or breakfast. Unlike a few years ago, we now have access to constantly available entertainment. When I was a teenager, after the 10 o'clock news there was little of interest on the TV… maybe an old film that was being replayed for what seemed like the hundredth time. Now, social media never sleeps, films and series are instantly streamed onto our TVs, laptops, and phones, and all of this has an impact on our sleep.

What is the Function of Sleep?

We spend about one-third of our life sleeping. Clearly, from an evolutionary perspective, it follows that sleep has to be of vital importance, and we now know that sleep is *as essential* as food and water to our survival. If we were in the business of torture, we would probably have sleep deprivation on our list of potential torture weapons. We would do this for a good reason; humans cannot survive for very long without sleep.

Randy Gardner is believed by many to have set the record for being the person who managed to stay awake for the longest period of time without sleep. When he was a teenager, he managed to stay awake for eleven days! In turn, it has been shown that after just three or four nights without sleep, people can start to hallucinate.

We know that sleep affects almost every tissue and system in the body. It affects the heart and brain. It impacts our metabolism, immune function, and mood.

Let's look at some of the benefits associated with adequate sleep.

Improved Memory, Concentration, and Learning

Every day, we encounter multiple stimuli and new pieces of information. Humans can't remember every aspect of what we experience, though. It is thought that when we sleep, we sort through and interpret all these experiences and memories. This helps us to make sense of, and memorise, important information.

Adequate sleep helps us improve our attention and learning, and it aids us in our decision making. Unsurprisingly, it has been shown that people who have not had enough sleep can have difficulties making decisions and solving problems.

Reduction in Toxins and Reduced Risk of Cognitive Decline and Alzheimer's Disease

There is growing evidence for a close reciprocal relationship between sleep disorders and cognitive decline. This means that there may be a connection between suffering from a sleep disorder and developing an illness such as Alzheimer's disease. It is thought that sleep helps us get rid of toxins that occur in the brain during normal activity; it helps us 'spring clean' the waste that we have produced in our body during the day.[14] Beta-amyloid is a protein that is associated with Alzheimer's disease. It is one of the toxins that get 'cleaned away' during sleep.[15]

Repair of Cells and Tissues in the Body

Deep sleep triggers the release of growth-promoting hormones, which boost muscle mass and repair cells and tissues in the body. We all know that babies sleep much of the day, much more than older children. It is perhaps not surprising that children's growth and development are linked with sleep. But because we may have stopped growing in height or shoe size, it does not mean that we don't need our sleep for the continued care and maintenance of our bodies.

Reduction in Risk of Becoming Overweight; Reduction in Risk of Developing Type 2 Diabetes and Cardiovascular Disease

Adequate sleep helps to maintain the balance of hormones in the body. When we don't sleep well, the levels of the hormone called leptin can fall. This hormone helps us feel full after eating. At the same time, when we have not had adequate sleep, we produce more of the hormone ghrelin. This hormone stimulates hunger. It is obvious that if the hormones that regulate the feeling of hunger and fullness are not adequately balanced, we can experience the desire to overeat and to crave sugary and unhealthy foods. This explains why chocolate and cake call out to many of us, demanding to be eaten when we haven't slept well!

It is thought that if people sleep for only five to six hours a night, they eat on average three hundred more calories the next day. This

---

[14] Bubu, O. M., Brannick, M., Mortimer, J., Umasabor-Bubu, O., Sebastião, Y. V., Wen, Y., ... Anderson, W. M. (2016). Sleep, Cognitive impairment, and Alzheimer's disease: A Systematic Review and Meta-Analysis. *Sleep*, 40(1). doi: 10.1093/sleep/zsw032.

[15] Xie, L., Kang, H., Xu, Q., Chen, M. J., Liao, Y., Thiyagarajan, M., ... Nedergaard, M. (2013). Sleep Drives Metabolite Clearance from the Adult Brain. *Science*, 342(6156), 373–377. doi: 10.1126/science.1241224.

can explain the link between inadequate sleep and levels of obesity.

Another important hormone in our body is insulin. Insulin is responsible for the regulation of glucose in the blood. There is evidence that inadequate sleep is associated with insulin resistance. Increased insulin resistance is associated with Type 2 Diabetes and cardiovascular disease.

Heart attacks occur most often on Monday mornings. Research has shown a 24% increase in the number of heart attacks on one particular Monday in the year, the Monday in Spring after the clocks go forward for daylight saving after we have typically lost an hour's sleep.[16] It is thought that people who are already vulnerable to heart disease may be more at risk after sudden time changes.

Increased Motivation to Exercise

It has been shown that when people don't have adequate levels of sleep, their motivation to engage in physical exercise is decreased. This is not unpredictable; who wants to go for a walk or swim when they are exhausted? But this can also present a catch-22; exercise can make you sleep better, and a lack of exercise can make it harder to fall asleep, after which you are tired, and don't want to do any exercise, and so on. On the flip side, breaking this cycle can be a very positive thing, as I will discuss in more detail later.

Better Immune System

It has been shown that people who have adequate levels of sleep have an immune system that functions better.[17]

We know that when we are unwell, our need for sleep increases. Think of the last time that you were unwell with the flu – your

---

[16] Sandhu, A., Seth, M., & Gurm, H. S. (2014). Daylight savings time and myocardial infarction. *Open Heart*, 1(1). doi: 10.1136/openhrt-2013-000019.

[17] Besedovsky, L., Lange, T., & Born, J. (2011). Sleep and immune function. *Pflügers Archiv - European Journal of Physiology*, 463(1), 121–137. doi: 10.1007/s00424-011-1044-0.

body craved sleep, and this sleep helped your immune system fight the virus.

Increased Energy

Many people with persistent pain struggle with low levels of energy. You don't need me to tell you that decreased energy levels are associated with inadequate levels of sleep. When you are able to improve your sleep, you will often find that your energy levels increase too.

Better Mental Health

Psychologists talk a lot about vicious circles, when one negative thing leads to another, and that leads to another, and so on. We know that a vicious circle exists when we consider sleep and mental health.

In the previous chapters, I outlined how stress, anxiety, and depression can all cause sleep difficulties. And it works the other way too – we know that inadequate sleep also impacts negatively on our mental health. I am sure that you have noticed how, even if your mental health is good, a poor night's sleep can impact on your mood the next day. If your sleep is persistently poor, it may have a significant impact on your mental health. Inadequate sleep is associated with depression, suicidal ideation (or thoughts of suicide), and even suicide attempts.

A lack of adequate sleep has also been shown to be associated with stress. During the deep sleep phase of sleep, your nervous system quietens down and your heart rate and blood pressure drop. The level of the stress hormone cortisol also decreases. Restoring our sleeping patterns can bring back this much-needed period of deep sleep.

Reduced Levels of Inflammation

It is believed that poor sleep is linked with increased levels of inflammation.[18] This is important because it is thought that there is a link between persistent pain and chronic inflammation.

The Mechanisms that Help your Body get to Sleep

Two biological mechanisms regulate your sleep. Circadian rhythms direct a wide range of functions in your body, from wakefulness to body temperature. They play a role in the timing of sleep, causing you to feel sleepy at night and causing you to wake in the morning.

In turn, sleep-wake homeostasis keeps track of your need to sleep. The homeostatic sleep drive reminds your body to sleep after a certain time. It also regulates sleep intensity. The drive to sleep becomes stronger every hour that you are awake.

Many factors influence your sleep-wake needs. Factors like stress, your sleep environment, and what you eat and drink influences your sleep.

Medical conditions and persistent pain influence sleep as do other factors like the medication we might be taking. We know that one of the greatest factors that influences sleep is exposure to light. Specialised cells in the retinas of your eyes tell your brain whether it is day or night, and this can have a big influence on your sleep-wake cycle.

Persistent Pain and Sleep

As I stated a moment ago, the inability to sleep well is a common difficulty for people who live with persistent pain. People with persistent pain often find it difficult to fall asleep. Additionally, many people report that their sleep is disrupted by pain. Some

---

[18] Mullington, J. M., Simpson, N. S., Meier-Ewert, H. K., & Haack, M. (2010). Sleep loss and inflammation. *Best practice & research. Clinical endocrinology & metabolism*, 24(5), 775–784. doi:10.1016/j.beem.2010.08.014.

people state that while they appear to have no difficulties falling or staying asleep, they don't feel rested or restored after sleeping.

Research indicates that having a bad night's sleep can make you more sensitive to pain.[19] Many people tell me that if they experience a lot of pain today, their sleep will be poorer tonight. They also know that if they sleep badly, their pain will be worse the next day.[20]

Why are Pain and Sleep so Closely Linked?

You will remember from the chapter on understanding pain that when you live with persistent pain, your nervous system is more sensitive and active. To fall asleep, your nervous system needs to calm down. It is not hard to see why a person living with pain can often struggle to fall asleep.

When we fall asleep, we move through several stages of slumber, varying from light to deep sleep. Sleep can be broadly divided into Rapid Eye Movement (REM) sleep and non-REM sleep. Sleep cycles are repeated several times throughout the night, with a complete sleep cycle taking on average 90 to 110 minutes. The first sleep cycles each night have relatively short REM sleeps and long periods of deep sleep but, later in the night, the period of REM sleeps lengthen and the time spent in deep sleep decreases.

It is normal to wake briefly several times a night between sleep cycles, but many people will get up the following day and do not even realise that they have been awake. However, like Pauline in the example above, if you live with persistent pain, during such a brief period of being awake, you may notice your pain and you may then struggle to get back to sleep as a result.

[19] Sivertsen, B., Lallukka, T., Petrie, K. J., Steingrímsdóttir, Ó. A., Stubhaug, A., & Nielsen, C. S. (2015). Sleep and pain sensitivity in adults. *Pain*, 156(8), 1433–1439. doi: 10.1097/j.pain.0000000000000131.

[20] Kelly, G. A., Blake, C., Power, C. K., O'keeffe, D., & Fullen, B. M. (2011). The Association Between Chronic Low Back Pain and Sleep. *The Clinical Journal of Pain*, 27(2), 169–181. doi: 10.1097/ajp.0b013e3181f3bdd5.

How Much Sleep do I Need?

There is no magic number of sleep hours that an individual requires. The amount of sleep you need, as well as your sleep patterns, vary as you age. The need for sleep varies across people of the same age, too. Whatever the case, we know that adults generally need between seven and nine hours of sleep a night.

If you aim to get seven hours of sleep a night, you may go to bed at midnight thinking that when the alarm goes off at 7 am, you will have gotten enough sleep. However, it is important to remember to build in time to fall asleep. Therefore, if you are aiming to have seven hours of sleep, you may need seven and a half hours of 'sleep opportunity' in bed.

If you wake up feeling refreshed, and generally wake up spontaneously without an alarm clock, within about half an hour of your usual time, you are probably getting enough sleep. Additionally, if you usually fall asleep within 30 minutes of going to bed, there are probably no significant lifestyle factors that are preventing you from sleeping.

Medication and Sleep

Many people who live with persistent pain have been prescribed medication to help them with their sleep problems. It is recommended that even if you are using prescribed medication to help you sleep that you also incorporate the tips below into your daily routine.

Techniques for Overcoming Sleeping Difficulties

It is important to remember that even if you live with pain, there are many things that you can do to help improve your sleep.

The techniques that I describe below will help you if, like Gary in the example above, you struggle with falling asleep. They will also help you if you are like Pauline and struggle to get *back* to sleep after awakening during the night. I know that many people who live with persistent pain struggle to get to sleep *and* stay asleep, and these techniques will help if you are experiencing both of these difficulties.

It is unlikely that any of the tips below will have an *immediate* impact on your sleep. However, if you implement the following recommendations, you should find that your sleep will improve over time.

You may decide to focus on one or two of these tips initially, and then gradually implement more and more of them.

Set a Sleep Schedule

What is a sleep schedule? A sleep schedule essentially means that you go to bed at roughly the same time every night and get up at the same time every morning. This includes weekends. This is not easy to implement but can be particularly hard for someone who is living with persistent pain. Many people who live with pain describe horrendous sleep. People have told me that they toss and turn all night and that they might have only managed a few hours of relatively undisturbed sleep when the alarm goes off. If this is the case for you, it can be very hard to maintain a sleep routine and get up at your designated time, especially if you are not working due to your pain or if you don't have to get up at a set time in the morning.

> **If you want to retrain your body into sleeping well, setting a sleep schedule is an essential part of the picture.**

I wear a fitness tracker and one of the features it has is an alarm to remind me to prepare for sleep. Occasionally, in the evening, I am caught up in something and don't realise how late it is. When my tracker buzzes, it serves as a reminder that it is time to get ready for bed and this simple alarm helps me stick to my sleep schedule. It can be worth setting an alarm to remind you to start getting ready for bed if you think it will help with your bedtime schedule.

People often tell me that they take a short nap during the day and this can be helpful, especially if it assists you in developing a schedule of time for bed and a time for getting up. However, a lot of people have admitted to me that their daytime napping can turn into marathon sessions, perhaps napping for four or five hours every day. Be careful if this is the case for you. Prolonged naps are likely to impact on your night-time sleep.

People often also report that their prolonged daytime naps can impact negatively on their quality of life. They may find that they are missing out on doing important things in life, and they are moving away from their values due to their need for prolonged daytime sleep. Slowly shortening daytime naps, and sticking to a regular and not-too-late bedtime, will help you shift your sleeping pattern back to the night, with no more than a short nap (if needed) during the day.

Don't Stay in Bed Tossing and Turning

If you cannot sleep after about 20-25 minutes, leave the bedroom and go to another room. Sit in dim lighting, doing something restful like reading or listening to some music. It is best if you don't eat. When you feel sleepy, return to bed. This tip is important because we know that the brain likes to make associations between two or more stimuli and that these associations can be very powerful. For example, I always associate going to the cinema with having popcorn, and as a result, it is very hard for me to resist popcorn when I go watch a movie!

If you have spent night after night tossing and turning in bed, your brain will begin to associate your bed with tossing and turning, making it less likely that you will sleep well. This tip is also challenging to implement; it is hard to get out of a warm, comfortable bed. However, it really does work for people who persist with it.

When we consider this tip, it is important to remember that it is not helpful to clock watch. How many times have you laid in bed, tossing and turning, watching the hours ticking by, panicking about your inability to sleep and worrying about how you are going to cope the next day? You might ask, "How will I know when twenty or twenty-five minutes have passed if I am not supposed to look at the clock?" Even without a clock, you will have a good idea when about twenty minutes have passed.

It is my experience that people often resist the advice regarding clock watching; it is as if they need to know how much time they have put into trying to fall asleep. I can recall one patient who slept very badly. It emerged that she had a special clock that projected the time on the ceiling in massive, red numbers! It constantly taunted her throughout the night, and every time she checked the time, she felt more and more anxious as the minutes ticked by and she still hadn't slept. When she removed this clock from her room, she found it easier to relax and go to sleep.

Keep your Bedroom for Sleep

Many people use their bedroom as a home office, a sitting room, or even a dining room. People often eat in bed, watch TV in bed, scroll through social media on their phone or work on their laptop in bed. These actions are not helpful for a variety of reasons. If you associate your bed with watching TV, no matter how relaxing that feels, it will make you less likely to sleep well. Similarly, if you work in bed, you are going to be less likely to associate your bed with sleep.

Take Electronics out of the Bedroom

This step can be difficult to implement, simply because we are all so attached to our TVs, phones, tablets and laptops. When I suggest that people remove their devices from the bedroom, I have been met with a lot of resistance. You won't be surprised when I tell you that I also meet a lot of resistance when I suggest this to my teenage children, as well! However, the removal of electronic devices – and limiting their use before bed – is one of the most crucial things we can do to help our sleep improve.

A number of my close friends are secondary school teachers, and they tell me what a difference they have noticed in their pupils since smartphones have become commonplace. They say that many pupils are now coming to school looking pale, drawn, and exhausted, and that their concentration is poor. They are certain it is because young people are spending hours on their phone when they are in bed, and they are not getting the rest that they need.

Before I discuss this further, I think it is worth taking an evolutionary perspective and thinking again about the lives that our ancestors lived. When humans lived in caves and small huts, they typically spent the last hours before bed, sitting in the dark with only a fire or a torch to light their way. As they sat in the relative darkness, perhaps chatting to friends and family, the melatonin levels in their brains increased. Melatonin is a hormone that helps us to sleep.

We know that electronic devices – like smartphones and tablets – emit blue light. This so-called blue light has the same wavelength of light as the morning sun. This 'morning light' that is coming from our electronic devices reduces the amount of melatonin produced. Is it any wonder that we struggle to go to sleep when we go to bed? Our prehistoric brains think it is time to get up and start hunting and gathering.

Aside from taking electronic devices out of the bedroom, what else can we do? Ideally, you would not watch TV or use your smartphone or tablet for about ninety minutes before bed. If limiting the use of your smartphone or tablet before bed is too difficult, you can consider downloading an app on your phone that limits the amount of blue light emitted from your screen. You might also consider buying amber glasses which cut out blue light wavelengths. They can be purchased relatively cheaply online.

Finally, try not to use your phone as your alarm clock. If you have your phone in the bedroom, there is always the temptation to look at it; there is evidence that even a quick look at your phone can disrupt the production of melatonin.

Develop a Sleep Routine

When I became a mother for the first time, I was desperate for my baby to sleep through the night. My mother's advice was to try to get my baby into a good sleep routine. It was good advice and it worked well.

As my babies grew into toddlers, I continued with a bedtime routine: a bath about half an hour before bed, changing into pyjamas, a story in bed using the soft light of the bedside lamp.

This routine worked; even before they could talk, they seemed to know the routine and quickly settled at night. This routine was occasionally disrupted if someone came to visit, and my youngsters always struggled to settle down for the night when their routine was disrupted.

Adults are not all that different to toddlers when it comes to bedtime routines. In the time before bed, a sleep routine will serve as a prompt to your subconscious mind – signalling that it is time for bed. Some people find that a warm bath or shower is a relaxing part of their bedtime routine, too. It is helpful as it increases the body surface temperature initially, followed by cooling; our core body temperature falls as we drop off to sleep.

If you enjoy reading, you might find it helpful to spend some time doing so before bed. Other people find burning lavender oil a helpful part of their bedtime routine. Ultimately, whatever bedtime routine you choose will involve activities that you routinely do before bed that help you relax and prepare for sleep.

If you reflect on your night-time routine, you might notice that some of the things you do cause you to feel upset or stressed. I used to watch the news before I went to bed but noticed that I frequently became emotional or upset. As a result, I decided to stop watching the news before bed and to spend time watching something lighter or reading before bed.

It can be helpful to avoid other potentially stressful activities before bed. Even checking emails in the hour before bed can impact negatively on our sleep. In the chapter on managing stress and anxiety, I talked about the culture of constant availability that has developed. If we use technology in the evening before bed, it can be very hard for our brains to slow down. We can feel pressured to respond to emails as soon as they come in, to comment on social media posts as soon as they are posted, and to answer texts as soon as they are received. If we engage in these tasks close to bedtime, our ability to relax and sleep well can be impacted.

Keep your Bedroom as Dark as Possible and Try to Stay Away from Bright Light Before Bed

As I explained above, melatonin is the hormone that is largely responsible for helping us sleep. Darkness encourages the production of melatonin. Therefore, it is a good idea to turn off bright lights at least ninety minutes before bed and to use sidelights or dimmed lights instead. It is also worth buying blackout blinds and/or blackout curtain linings for your bedroom. This can help you fall asleep and stay asleep, especially in the summer when it is only dark for a few hours.

Spend Time Outside Every Morning If Possible

Let's consider our ancestors' experience again. When the sun came up, they got up and started their day, making the most of the sunlight. We are designed to go outside into the sunlight. In a previous chapter, I talked about the benefits of sunlight for our mental health.

> # Getting outside and having exposure to sunlight also helps us sleep.

This applies whether we live in a country where the sun is frequently shining or somewhere where the sky is frequently grey and cloudy. It is important to get outside, and the greatest benefits are attained by getting out in *morning* sunlight (without sunglasses). Many people with pain spend long periods of time indoors. I have met very many people who rarely leave their homes, perhaps only going somewhere outside their homes a couple of times a week. I am convinced that this lack of time outdoors has a negative impact on their mental health and their sleep.

It can be difficult to spend time outside if you are in pain and particularly if the weather is poor. People have successfully incorporated more outdoor time into their lives by taking their dog out for a walk, or by sitting outside to have a cup of tea (well wrapped up if necessary), or by walking to the corner shop instead of taking the car.

Don't Take Caffeine After Lunch

As touched upon previously, caffeine is one of my favourite treats in life; there is nothing better than a good cup of coffee. However, caffeine is a substance that has a very long half-life. The half-life of a drug refers to how long it takes for the initial effect to reduce by 50%.

We know that the half-life of caffeine is approximately 6-7 hours, depending on a person's genetic make-up. This means that if you have a coffee at 6 pm and you go to bed at midnight, about half of the caffeine that was in the cup of coffee is still swilling around your brain at 12 o'clock. Interestingly, caffeine also has a long quarter-life (approximately twelve hours). Therefore, a quarter of the caffeine that was in that cuppa that you had at noon is still in your system at midnight.

I often get funny looks from friends if I go out for dinner and decline a cup of coffee after the meal. They know that I love coffee, and they often tell me how lucky they are that caffeine never stops *them* from sleeping. Even if you think that you are like some of my friends, and reckon that caffeine doesn't impact your sleep, it is important to remember that caffeine also impacts on the *quality of your sleep*, reducing your capacity to experience deep sleep.

Coffee has a bad reputation when it comes to caffeine, but it is important to consider how tea, green tea, and some soft drinks also contain caffeine, so-called energy drinks especially.

If I am having a coffee in the afternoon, I will switch to decaffeinated coffee. Decaffeinated coffee still contains some caffeine, though; as much as 20% of conventional coffee, depending on the brand. Many people have told me that they find non-caffeinated herbal tea a good substitute for coffee and tea in the afternoon and evening.

Recognise the Impact of Alcohol on Sleep

People often use alcohol to help them sleep; if you have chronic difficulty with sleep, it is all too easy to rely on alcohol to help yourself drop off. It is very true that if you drink enough, you will fall asleep, but one of the difficulties associated with using alcohol to aid sleep – just as with caffeine – is that it affects the quality of your sleep. When people have been drinking, they wake more often during the night. While they might not remember waking up during the night, the next morning, they do report that they don't feel refreshed, even if their drinking was not excessive.

We also know that alcohol affects our sleep cycles. REM is a phase of sleep that is critical for emotional processing. When people have been drinking, their REM sleep is affected.

Consider the Temperature of your Bedroom

We sleep better in cooler environments. It has been found that the optimal room temperature for sleep is 18°.

Become More Active During the Day

Yes, we are back to this old chestnut – physical activity and exercise having many benefits. Better sleep is yet another benefit of increasing your activity levels. Within the hour or two before you plan to go to sleep, it is best not to engage in any vigorous exercise, as it causes your heartbeat to increase and your body to sweat. Gentle stretching before bed is fine, though.

Practise Mindfulness Meditation

As I have stated previously, there is good evidence that the regular practice of mindfulness meditation helps improve sleep. Many people have told me that they have noticed a significant improvement in their sleep after a relatively short period of practising mindfulness meditation. It is important to remember that even if you meditate in the morning, it can help you sleep at night. However, people often find that incorporating bedtime meditation into their bedtime routine can help them quieten their minds and prepare for sleep.

Cope with a Racing Mind

There are times when I struggle to sleep due to a racing mind. I go to bed, and just as I am getting comfortable, my mind starts to rev up. Typically, I think about some of the things that happened earlier in the day and some of the things that I have planned and need to remember for the next day. I know that a racing mind is a common difficulty for people. One way I have of managing this, is to keep a notebook and pen on my bedside locker. If I am beginning to fall asleep and suddenly remember that I have forgotten to send an important email, I will find it hard to switch my mind off. However, if I make a quick note of it in my notebook (often done without switching the light on), I know that it is there for me to pick up in the morning. That way, I can forget about it until morning. This is a good tip if you find that your mind is racing with things that you need to remember.

We have touched upon how our minds are very good at looking for danger and telling us scary stories. If we have difficulty sleeping, our minds can be very good at getting hooked into the story of how bad this is, how fatigued we will be the next day, etc. etc. If you notice that you are getting caught up in these stories while lying in bed, use the techniques already described for coping with these stories.

You can direct your attention to physical sensations; for example, notice the parts of your body in contact with the bed. Alternatively, you can rest your attention on your breath by paying close attention to breathing in, noticing the pause, noticing breathing out, and paying attention to the pause, before you take another breath.

Practise your Breathing

In the chapter on anxiety and stress, I described several different breathing techniques that help manage anxiety and stress. These techniques are useful to relax your body before bed, or in bed if you notice that you are feeling anxious or if your body is tense. The 4-7-8 or 3-4-5 breathing techniques (see Chapter 8) are particularly helpful.

Avoid Heavy, Fatty or Sugary Foods Before Bed

If you can, try to avoid fatty or sugary foods before bed, and try to eat before 7 pm if possible. This will allow your body some time to digest your food before you go to sleep.

Things to Remember

- Sleep is essential for our physical and psychological wellbeing.

- Adequate sleep has many benefits, including improved memory, concentration, and learning, reduced risk of being overweight and developing cardiovascular diseases, plus an improved immune system and better mental health.

- Many people with persistent pain struggle to sleep well. Research indicates that a bad night's sleep can make you more sensitive to pain.

- There are many techniques that you can use to help improve your sleep. Find which work best for you!

CHAPTER 12: EAT WELL AND MANAGE EMOTIONAL EATING

> ## Food can fuel your body or feed your emotions

All of us know that an unhealthy diet can cause us to gain weight, and – in our culture – we seem to be obsessed with looking good. In most women's magazines, there will be at least one article on how to lose weight and look more attractive. Often, there will be a picture of a celebrity on the front cover who is being vilified for putting on weight, or who is promoting some new miracle diet. But while a poor diet is associated with weight gain, we often forget that a poor diet is also linked to poor physical *and* mental health. Therefore, I don't think any book on pain management would be complete without a chapter on eating well.

People often tell me that they find the information about diet and nutrition confusing. For example, a few years ago, we were told that eating too many eggs was bad for us, and now the NHS guidelines suggest that there should be no limit on the number of eggs that we eat. One of the reasons for these conflicting messages is that science and research into nutrition continue to evolve. While the jury is still out on several issues within the field of nutrition, some basic guidelines are now well established. We should all try to follow them to ensure that we maintain good physical and mental health.

Over the years, discussions about diet have consistently come up in my consultations with people who live with persistent pain. Many people have told me that their diet has deteriorated since they developed their pain. A significant number of people that I meet are upset by the weight that they have gained since they developed their pain.

When you are sore and in pain, you want comfort, and you might crave something – anything– to ease your distress. One of the easiest ways to comfort ourselves is by choosing something that is readily and cheaply available – food.

I have used food to comfort myself. At times, when I have had a hard day, if I am feeling upset or if I am bored, I have engaged in comfort or emotional eating. I have eaten food that has provided me with a brief high; for me, that food is usually chocolate and sweet treats. I think that there are very few people who have never engaged in emotional eating. For people with persistent pain, the need for a bit of comfort can lead to more regular emotional eating and a tendency to resort to eating sweet or unhealthy snacks as a way of lifting one's mood a little.

On the other hand, some people who live with pain may struggle to eat. This can be due to the side effects of medication, or it can be because they are depressed and their appetite is poor. They may rely on snacks to keep going, and these snacks often don't provide the nutrition that their bodies need to function.

Many people have also told me that they have struggled to cook since they developed their pain. They might struggle to chop vegetables or lift heavy saucepans. As a result, they have become more reliant on convenience foods that require minimal preparation; foods that are easy to put in the oven or microwave.

Several medications that are prescribed to manage pain can stimulate the appetite and lead to weight gain. We also know that most people who develop persistent pain become increasingly inactive. These two factors can lead to people gaining weight, and this increase can have a significant negative impact on self-esteem.

I am going to break this chapter into two sections. In the first section, I will provide you with some basic information about the components of a healthy diet and provide you with tips on improving your diet. I am *not* a dietician or nutritionist, and this information is very general. I advise you to consult your family doctor or a qualified dietician for specific dietary advice.

In the second section of the chapter, I will provide you with some tips on managing emotional eating.

Tips for Improving Your Diet

Drink More Fluids

It is believed that the majority of people don't drink enough water, and that they are frequently dehydrated without knowing so. About 60% of the body is made up of water. We can only live for a few days without it. Many people who live with persistent pain complain about feeling tired all the time. It is known that dehydration contributes to difficulties with fatigue. If you regularly experience fatigue, try to increase your daily intake of water to see if this may help.

Constipation is a side-effect of some pain medications, and unfortunately, it is often one of the side effects that does not resolve when your body adjusts to the medication. Dehydration contributes to difficulties with constipation, so if this is an issue for you, explore whether drinking more fluids might help you.

Dehydration can also contribute to the development of headaches and make skin conditions worse.

If sugar cravings are an issue for you, it is worth knowing that when you are well hydrated, your sugar cravings will reduce.

How Much Fluid Should You Drink Every Day?

While there are no hard and fast rules, it is recommended that most people should aim to drink approximately 2 litres of fluids a day; this equates to approximately eight medium glasses of water. If you live somewhere hot, you will have to increase your fluid intake above that level. If drinking 2 litres seems unrealistic for you, try to drink at least 1.2 litres of water which equates to about 8 small glasses of water a day.

People often use their thirst as a guide for their need to drink more liquids, but did you know that if you are thirsty, you are already dehydrated? Even if you are not thirsty, you may still be dehydrated. Use the colour of your urine to monitor your hydration levels. If you are well-hydrated, your urine should be a pale colour; darker coloured urine indicates that you are dehydrated.

What Should You Drink?

Water is a great way to increase your fluids, and it is recommended that the majority of your fluid intake should be made up of water.

Tea and coffee can be included in your fluid intake. However, it is worth being mindful of how much caffeine you drink every day. I talked about caffeine in the chapter on sleep, and many nutritionists recommend that we restrict our coffee intake to 1 or 2 cups of coffee a day, and our tea intake to 3 or 4 cups per day. Many people like to take herbal tea as an alternative hot drink to tea and coffee.

Most nutritionists advise that we avoid drinking artificially sweetened drinks as much as possible. While there does not appear to be any definitive evidence that consuming artificially sweetened drinks is bad for your health, there are some studies that have shown a correlation or relationship between drinking zero-calorie soft drinks and the development of diabetes.

Throughout my career, I have met many diet drink addicts; people who drink multiple diet drinks every day. The patients I know who decided to cut down on the number of these drinks *all* reported feeling better after doing so. Cutting down on soft drinks can be difficult, particularly if you drink a lot of them. Try replacing one with a glass of water or a cup of tea every day, and slowly reduce the number of soft drinks. If you do manage to break the habit, your taste buds will get the opportunity to change and the drinks will taste different after a few weeks.

If you want to lose weight, it is important to remember that many drinks contain large numbers of calories. Sugary drinks are full of so-called 'empty calories' that can contribute to a quick high, followed by a slump in energy levels. It is also important to remember that certain hot drinks, milkshakes, smoothies, and the like, may also contain large numbers of calories. I can recall one lady telling me that she was actively trying to lose weight and that when she met her friend for coffee a couple of times a week, she made sure to stick to coffee and not snack on sweet treats. She told me that she typically drank a large vanilla latte. When we researched the calories contained in the drink, she was shocked to find that it was nearly 400(!); the average woman consumes about 2,000 calories a day to maintain a healthy weight. That one coffee contained a fifth of the recommended calorie intake for an average woman.

Suggestions to Help You Increase Your Fluid Intake

Consider adding some fruit to your water. It can be challenging to drink a lot of water, particularly during the winter when it is cold. Adding fruit to the water can help; slices of lemon, orange, or berries are great for adding some flavour to water.

Try using a water bottle. Many people find it useful to carry a water bottle around with them – even when they are at home – so that they can continually sip at water throughout the day. I always have a water bottle sitting on my desk, and I find myself sipping water without even realising it.

Try to drink a glass of water about half an hour before eating. When we are establishing new habits, it can be helpful to anchor them onto existing habits to help them 'stick'. You are likely to eat a meal at least three times a day and if you get into the habit of drinking a glass of water before each of those meals, you will automatically increase your fluid intake. In addition, numerous studies have shown that drinking a glass of water about 30 minutes before eating can result in the person feeling fuller, thereby consuming fewer calories at those meals. This habit could therefore help with weight loss if that is something that you are interested in.

Drink water between meals. If you are hungry between meals, try drinking a glass of water as we often mistake dehydration for feelings of hunger.

Eat More Fruit and Vegetables

In the UK, it is recommended that we eat at least 5 portions of fruit and vegetables a day. Most of us know about this, but it is often difficult to implement this advice. Many people find it easier to eat fruit than vegetables; eating fruit is quick and easy and typically needs no preparation. While fruits, and particularly berries, are very good for us, it is important to try to include as many vegetables in our diet as possible.

Vegetables are full of vitamins, minerals, nutrients, phytonutrients, and fibre, and it is known that green, leafy vegetables are particularly good for us. Nutritionists advise us to try to 'eat the rainbow' – meaning that we should try to eat vegetables of different colours. It is known that plant-based fibre is especially beneficial. Eating plenty of this fibre can help reduce inflammation, something that can be particularly helpful for someone living with persistent pain. It is believed that brightly-coloured fibre-rich vegetables like carrots, broccoli, spinach, red onion, asparagus, and olives can also help regulate blood sugar control, reduce blood pressure, improve cardiovascular health and improve immune function.

When I recently had a discussion with my son about the importance of including enough fruit and vegetables in his diet, he tried to convince me that drinking a couple of glasses of fruit juice equates to two portions of fruit. Unfortunately, we know that drinking fruit juice does not provide the same benefits as eating the fruit. The fibre has been removed from fruit juice, and a glass of fruit juice can contain very high levels of sugar; one glass of orange juice has as much sugar as a glass of soda.

Reduce the Amount of Processed Food You Eat

As I said previously, many people seem to increase the amount of processed food they eat since developing their pain. I can completely understand this. If you are sore and lacking in energy, it can be hard to get the motivation to prepare a healthy meal, particularly if you are living on your own, or do not have to prepare a meal for other family members.

Let's discuss the downsides of processed foods. I firmly believe if a miracle happened, and processed food was removed from the world, our physical and mental health would improve dramatically.

What is Processed Food?

The easiest way to work out if a food is processed or not is to take a quick look at the food label. If it contains more than 5 ingredients, it is likely to be a 'processed' food. Additionally, if the ingredients contain foodstuffs that you don't recognise – with words that are difficult to pronounce – or ingredients that are a group of letters and numbers, it is likely to be processed.

Most processed foods are energy or calorie-dense, and they are usually high in sugar, salt, and the types of fat that are known to be unhealthy. Also, they are often a poor source of protein, fibre, and micronutrients, which are the things that we should be looking for in food. When you eat a lot of processed food, it is easy to eat more than the recommended levels of sugar, salt, and fat, as it is unclear how much of this has been added to the food.

In recent years there has been a lot of interest in so-called 'anti-inflammatory diets'. Typical inflammatory foods are processed foods with low nutritional value. It is known that inflammation plays a key role in many of the chronic health conditions that people are living with, and it is thought that a lot of persistent pain is the result of chronic inflammation. There is good evidence that chronic inflammation can be *reduced* by making dietary changes. Reducing or avoiding processed foods is a very good place to start if you want to improve your diet and especially if you want to try to reduce inflammation.

When we think about inflammation, there are not only things to avoid, there are also things to try to eat more of. Antioxidants, for example, have anti-inflammatory effects. Some fruits – like red grapes, blueberries, and cherries – contain antioxidants that have been shown to reduce inflammatory pain.

You may want to research anti-inflammatory diets in more detail. But if you want to keep it simple, you can assume that a varied diet, containing plenty of vegetables and fruit, which does not include processed food, is likely an anti-inflammatory diet.

Reduce the Amount of Sugar in Your Diet

The vast majority of us (and I include myself in this) eat too much sugar. We are programmed to love sugar. However, it was not meant to be a staple part of our diet. In caveman times, whilst sweet fruit was occasionally available, often at the end of the summer, sugar was not readily available. Our bodies craved this sweet food that was rarely available, because consumption of it allowed us to lay down fat for tough times when food was not so plentiful.

These days, we no longer live in 'feast or famine' times, and chocolate brownies are available to us across all four seasons of the year! However, our craving for sugar hasn't become extinct; we are challenged to manage it every day.

We know that sugar is addictive. When we consume sugar, a part of our brain associated with pleasure, reward, and addiction is activated. This is the same area of the brain that is activated when people use nicotine, cocaine, and heroin. Is it any wonder that we find it hard to ignore that chocolate bar calling when we are sore, tired, or upset?

Too much sugar can cause weight gain. This is very obvious but is still worth stating. We know that rates of obesity are rising throughout the world, and it is believed that sugar – in drinks and food – is one of the main reasons for this. Being overweight or obese is associated with many physical consequences, including feeling very tired, feeling breathless, and having difficulties doing physical activity. If you are living with persistent pain, you probably already experience difficulties with fatigue and physical activity, and being overweight can add to these.

Many people who are overweight have talked to me about the significant impact that their weight has had on their self-esteem. Often their self-esteem is low anyway due to their pain. Their weight further adds to their difficulties with self-esteem.

Whilst we are aware that we are eating sugary food, we typically underestimate just *how much* sugar the food contains. When I bake sweet treats, I am always shocked at the amount of sugar that is part of the ingredient list. It is easy to see a small chocolate brownie sitting on a shelf in the café and not to appreciate the amount of sugar that it contains.

When we eat that brownie, it is obvious to us that we are eating something that contains sugar. However, we often eat sugar without even realising it. Take bread, for example, which is a staple in most of our diets. Years ago, bread contained only three ingredients: flour, water, and salt. Nowadays, most loaves of bread have sugar added to them. In turn, many processed foods, ready meals, and sauces (such as ketchup, mayonnaise, even salad dressing) have sugar added to them.

Reading food labels is one of the best ways to monitor your intake of added sugar. Be alert when the word sugar is not used in the ingredient list. Ingredients ending in "ose" like dextrose, fructose, glucose, sucrose and lactose, plus corn sugar and honey may be used instead.

Our gut and our gut's microflora (the bacteria that live in our gut that help us break down the foods we eat) play an important role in our health. A diet that is high in sugar can have a negative effect on the gut, which in turn harms our health. A diet high in sugar is associated with sugar cravings, low energy, poor concentration, and tiredness. These symptoms are very commonly described by the people I see who are living with persistent pain. When we feel like this, we are drawn to consume more sugar or refined carbohydrates (e.g., pasta, white bread, white rice). And so, the cycle of eating too much sugar continues.

When we consistently eat a diet that contains too much sugar, insulin resistance can occur. When your blood sugar can no longer be adequately controlled, you can be diagnosed with Type 2 Diabetes.

It has also been shown that sugar intake can increase levels of stress hormones like cortisol. Cortisol can contribute to sugar cravings, and stress can also contribute to difficulties with blood sugar regulation. So, we enter a vicious circle of stress and sugar cravings. We can add low mood into the circle too. We know that people who are depressed have low levels of the neurotransmitter serotonin. Studies have also shown that low levels of serotonin stimulate sugar cravings.

Okay, okay – too much sugar is bad!

How Much Sugar Should We Consume Per Day?

The UK's NHS recommends that sugar shouldn't take up more than 5% of our calorie intake. This is about 30g of sugar a day for adults.

It is hard to reduce our consumption of sugar, and I have included some advice about managing sugar cravings and making positive changes to our diet later in this chapter.

Include Protein in your Diet

Many people that I meet describe their diet as very carbohydrate-heavy, as they rely on easy to prepare foods, like toast or cereal, for more than one meal a day, particularly when they are having a flare-up of their pain or when they are very tired. Protein can form a very small part of their diet.

When we think of protein-rich foods, we often think of meat and fish, but many other foods are high in protein too. Beans, nuts, seeds, legumes (baked beans, lentils, etc.), and eggs are good foods to consider when trying to eat a diet that is rich in protein.

We know that protein is crucial for the growth and repair of tissues and the stabilisation of blood sugars that help us feel full. In the section on sugar, I described the vicious circle of sugar cravings and the quick fix that we can get from a sugary snack. We know that protein plays a key role in the stabilisation of blood sugars, and the incorporation of more protein in our diet can help us get out of the sugary vicious circle.

Nutritionists often recommend that we have three portions of protein a day, which might include one portion for breakfast, lunch, and dinner. It is worth bearing in mind that it is recommended that processed meat such as ham, bacon, and sausages should not be eaten too regularly.

Try to Eat a Diet Rich in Omega-3

Omega-3 is of particular interest to people living with persistent pain because it has been shown to have anti-inflammatory effects. For example, there is evidence that an increased intake of Omega-3 is associated with a reduction of inflammation which can cause swelling and pain.

Omega-3 is a so-called 'fatty acid'; it is an essential nutrient found in certain foods. In addition to its anti-inflammatory qualities, it is known that Omega-3 may play a role in stabilising mood, which is important when we consider our psychological wellbeing. Omega-3 may also help with difficulties with fatigue and memory.

Oily fish is very beneficial to our health as it is a good source of Omega-3. Fish rich in Omega-3 include anchovies, herring, salmon, mackerel, sardines, trout, and tuna. Omega-3 can also be found in flaxseed and flaxseed oil, chia seeds, walnuts, beans, eggs, kale, and spinach – so if you are vegetarian, you don't have to miss out. Omega-3 supplements are also available to buy.

It is important not to get confused between Omega-3 and Omega-6. Many vegetable oils, including soybean oil, contain high levels of Omega-6. Soybean oil is used in the production of many processed and fast foods. Omega-6 is known to be pro-inflammation. It is recommended that we have a good ratio of Omega-3 and Omega-6 in our diets. There is also evidence that in recent decades – as our diet has changed to include more processed foods – our dietary intake of Omega-6 has increased significantly. While we know that inflammation is necessary for survival, as it helps protect our body from infection and injury, it is thought that it can contribute to disease when it is excessive. Therefore, it may be worth considering whether you are getting enough Omega-3 in your diet and whether you may benefit from reducing your levels of Omega-6 by decreasing the amount of processed or fast food you are eating.

Simple Strategies Can Help You Manage Emotional Eating

Now that we have looked at some of the components of a healthy diet, it is important to consider the strategies that can help us make positive changes to our diet and manage emotional eating.

Work Out Your 'Why'

We have talked about this before, but you must consider the reasons *why* you want to make changes to your life – in this case, *why* you want to make changes to your diet and eating.

It is hard to make changes to diet; all of us are drawn to stay within our comfort zones, to repeat old habits endlessly. Our default setting is to do what we have always done.

If you are clear about your 'why', you are much more likely to make the changes that you need to improve your diet.

Here is a short exercise for you to try. Take out your notebook once more, and do the following:

Write down your reasons behind why you want to make changes to your diet. It is best to frame these reasons positively; for example, it is better to write down "I want to have more energy" rather than "I want to stop feeling so tired all the time."

Write down all the reasons that you can think of – some of them may be related to your health, and some of them may be related to your body image or self-confidence.

Make your list strong and inspiring. Include things to aim for, but remain realistic.

It can be helpful to keep your list of 'whys' somewhere prominent where you can read them often, preferably every day. I know people who have kept a list of their reasons for change on their phone, and set an alarm to remind them to read their reasons every day.

Plan Ahead

Any professional who helps people improve their diet will stress the importance of planning. You want to plan what you are going to eat, when you are going to buy your food, and when you are going to prepare your food. This planning can make it much more likely that you will be able to improve your diet.

When we consider the situation for people who live with persistent pain, it is *even more important* that they plan their diet and eat healthier every day. You will be very aware that flare-ups seem to happen out of the blue and all your plans for that day, or a few days in a row, may have to be modified or even completely abandoned. As a result, it can be helpful to ensure that you have something healthy – that is easy to prepare or heat up – close to hand, as there will be the temptation to reach for unhealthy snacks or meals during these times.

Keeping frozen vegetables in the house at all times can be helpful. They are healthy, make life easy, and don't need to be washed or chopped whether you are experiencing a flare-up or not.

Many people also find it helpful to batch cook some meals and freeze them. This way, you have something to quickly heat up if you are in a lot of pain, short on time, or low in energy.

A slow cooker is a great, relatively inexpensive addition to a kitchen. You can add your ingredients quickly and then just turn it on and forget about it while a healthy meal is cooked slowly.

Try to become familiar with a few simple, healthy meals that are quick and easy to prepare. They can come in useful for those days when you are feeling very sore or fatigued and don't have the energy to plan a healthy meal.

Removing unhealthy food from the house is also a good idea. If you don't have any cakes or crisps in the cupboard, it is less likely that you will go to the bother of leaving the house to get some.

Consider What Your Mind Has to Say About Eating

You know by now that your mind is constantly chattering and that some of the chatter is helpful in that it helps you move towards your values. You also know that some of that chatter is unhelpful and that it has the potential to move you away from the things that are important to you and give meaning to your life.

Your mind may say things to you like, "You are overweight because everyone in your family is overweight, there is nothing you can do about it" or "You have too much to cope with, there is no point in trying to improve your diet." If you can develop the capacity to observe your thoughts and listen to your mind's chatter, you can then decide whether you want to listen to the directions of your mind.

Remember that your mind is primed to tell you things that will keep you within your comfort zone. I have said it before, and I will say it again, your mind is trying to keep you safe and alive; it doesn't care if you are happy and living a fulfilled life.

> **Your mind is likely to come up with many different and very plausible reasons why you can't make changes to your diet.**

To manage this, you can remember that you have the freedom and the power to observe your mind's chatter, to observe its urges, and

195

to decide whether you want to listen to the chatter or give in to the urges.

Remember That Small Changes Count

I can recall one of my patients, let's call her Sophie, who wanted to improve her diet and lose some weight. She told me that periodically she declared, "That's it – I am cutting way back on my food and I am only going to eat healthy, very low-calorie food, like salads and vegetables." She usually skipped breakfast, ate a small green salad for lunch and a small dinner mainly consisting of vegetables. Can you imagine how long this new regimen lasted?

Sophie sometimes managed to get to Friday before she caved in and ordered a Chinese takeaway, washed it down with wine, and followed dinner up with a large bag of crisps in front of the TV. She typically went to bed on Friday night feeling guilty and angry with herself. She then adopted an all or nothing approach to her eating, saying things like, "I have ruined all my good work, I may as well eat what I want now." Sophie would typically go back to an unhealthy diet of processed and high sugar foods for a week or two until she declared that she had enough and began eating a very rigid, restricted diet. And, unsurprisingly, the rollercoaster continued month after month.

To break this cycle, I encouraged Sophie to change one or two small things first and then build upon that. Instead of eating a low-calorie, restricted diet, Sophie decided that she would try to eat at least one nutritious meal every day for a week. This went well for her, so then she decided to introduce a second nutritious meal every day the following week. Sophie felt that this was achievable and realistic. Finally, she aimed to eat three nutritious meals on most days.

When she was working on improving her diet, Sophie recognised that when she 'went on a diet', she was too rigid with her food, eating only very low-calorie food. In doing so, she didn't eat enough food to fuel her body. Sophie also began to appreciate that her 'all or nothing' approach to her diet wasn't helpful, and that if she did have a day when her diet was particularly unhealthy that she could adopt a more self-compassionate approach.

You *do not* have to radically change your diet overnight. Like Sophie, it can be helpful to plan smaller changes that you can implement over time.

Consider The Function of Food in Your Life

Food is used throughout the world as an expression of love – think of the meal that you cooked for your partner for a special occasion, or that box of chocolates on Valentine's Day. Sharing food with people you love is one of life's greatest pleasures and it is why so many of us greatly enjoy going out for a meal with family or friends.

As well as being an expression of love, food is universally used to comfort and alleviate distress. The vast majority of us will have been offered food to console us or to cheer us up. As a new mother, when my baby was distressed and crying, one of the first things I did was to offer him some milk, even if I wasn't sure that he was hungry. Given our experiences in our formative years, is it any wonder that we use food as a comfort?

> **There is nothing at all wrong with using food as an expression of love or for comfort. But what happens if food becomes your main way of showing love to yourself or comforting yourself? What happens if you often use food to manage your distress?**

As I said a moment ago, we know that when we are distressed and in need of comfort, we tend to reach for sugary and unhealthy foods; it seems that for the majority of us, carrots and celery sticks just do not provide the same comfort as a bar of chocolate or a bag of crisps.

I have illustrated a typical cycle of emotional eating below:

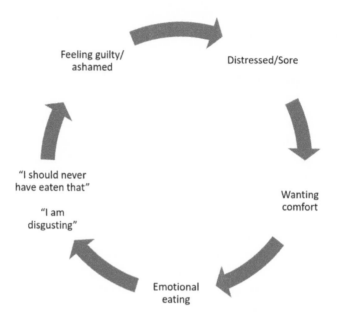

As you can see, it is a vicious circle. It starts with distress and wanting comfort, then followed by emotional eating. After the emotional eating, regret often sets in, followed by guilt and distress, and so on...

Distress is part of the human condition; it is something that you will encounter frequently. If you regularly use emotional eating as a way of alleviating your distress, you will find yourself in the kind of vicious circle, above, a lot of the time.

The first step in getting out of this vicious circle is to recognise when you are distressed. You may be feeling stressed, anxious, low in mood, lonely or bored. Many times, you may not be fully aware of how you are feeling. It is worth developing ways to recognise *when* you are distressed, or even *why* you are bored or lonely and comfort eating for those reasons. Then you can implement other ways of comforting and soothing yourself.

How Do You Recognise When You Are Distressed?

Regular practice of mindfulness meditation will help you become more aware – aware of your thoughts and your emotions.

Also, it can be helpful to pause before you eat something to recognise what you are feeling. Are you hungry? If you were to use a hunger scale from 0 to 10, where 10 is stuffed full and 0 is ravenously hungry, where would you be on that scale? Do you feel that hunger in your stomach, or do you feel an emotion in some other part of your body?

After you begin to tune into your body and your emotions, you may start to recognise patterns that you have developed. For example, you may notice that an argument with your partner triggers feelings of anger, frustration, and sadness. You may notice that you feel these emotions in your body; perhaps you detect tightness in your chest and an empty feeling in the pit of your stomach. You may notice that you want to push them away by eating, even though you are not hungry. If you manage to tune in, you can now choose to eat or do something different to comfort yourself. This is not always easy to accomplish, but even if you manage to do this some of the time, it will help you to free yourself from the vicious cycle of emotional eating.

I mentioned urges, above. An urge is when you have a strong desire or impulse to do something. It is normal to have urges to behave in a certain way, but we need to remember that always following our urges can lead us away from the life that we want to live. It is important to acknowledge that we can manage our urges; we can choose to give into them, or pay no attention.

> **Just like a surfer on a wave, we can choose to 'ride the urge' and let it pass.**

If I am late for a meeting and the road is clear, I might have the urge to speed to get to the meeting on time. I can give in to that urge or I can take a step back, observe the urge to speed, and choose a different path and stay within the speed limit.

If I have the urge to eat something sugary or unhealthy, I can develop the capacity to observe that urge. I can give in to it and eat the chocolate, or I can 'surf the urge' and let it pass. Observing the urge is not easy. I know that when I have the urge to eat something sugary, it is very hard to stand back and observe; I just want to dive into that chocolate! I am more likely to be able to 'surf the urge' if I can tune into my values, my 'whys', even if it is just for a moment. The beauty with urges is that like a wave, they don't last forever. They come and they go. Often when you distract yourself, you find that the urge subsides.

> **No matter how difficult it may seem, no matter how automatic the behaviour may appear, we can develop the capacity to choose something different from our usual response.**

What is the Function of Eating for You?

All behaviour has a function. If the function of food – for you – is *to alleviate your distress*, you need to develop what psychologists call 'functionally equivalent behaviour'. This essentially involves finding activities or behaviour that can serve the same function as food (alleviating distress), but which do not involve eating. In this way, food can return to its proper function in your life: to provide nourishment and keep you healthy.

> **If you have a repertoire of comforting activities available to you, you will no longer be so reliant on food to comfort you.**

If you engage in a lot of emotional eating and you want to do something about it, spend some time drawing up a list of things that you find relaxing and comforting; things that alleviate the inevitable distress that comes with being human. The list might include things like having a long bath, watching a movie or series on TV, having a massage, playing a game with your child, reading a good book, listening to your favourite music, chatting to a friend, going for a facial, going for a walk, petting your dog, asking for a hug, or reading a magazine. Some of the activities may cost money, but it is also important to choose activities that do not cost money and which are freely available to you if you need immediate comfort or if you need to relax.

It is my experience as a psychologist that many people never prioritise or give any thought to their need for 'self-soothing'. It is vital for everyone to make time for, and to engage in, self-soothing.

Get Family and Friends On Board

It is going to be very hard to make any changes to your diet if the people that you live with and/or friends are not on board with you. Have a conversation with your partner, family members, or friends about the changes that you would like to make to your diet and your reasons for making those changes.

A note of caution here – your family and friends may not be on the same page as you with this. They may not have a good appreciation of the importance of nutrition in physical and mental health or pain management. They may not have a good diet themselves and may not be ready to make changes to their own lives. They could see your intention to make changes as shining a spotlight on their poor diet and they may sabotage your efforts to change in a subconscious attempt to avoid dealing with their own dietary issues.

It is difficult if your friends and family are not supportive. You are going to have to accept that you can manage the direction of only one life – yours. You can only take responsibility for *your* health and ultimately it is every adult's responsibility to make their own choices about how they live their life. You can still move forward with your goals and try to get support where you can. Many online communities offer fantastic encouragement to people who are trying to make dietary changes to improve their health.

Eat Mindfully

Have you ever eaten a bag of crisps or sweets and been astonished to find that you have finished the bag already? I know I have. Often, when this has happened to me, I have been doing something else at the same time as eating – perhaps scrolling on my phone, watching TV, or working on my computer. I mindlessly put my hand into the bag, only to find the bag empty. This mindless eating is a sure way to overeat. How can we counteract this?

> **There is good evidence that mindful eating can help us manage emotional eating and adopt a healthier diet.**

If you think that you want to try to eat more mindfully, there are a couple of steps that you can follow.

When you are eating, try not to engage in any other distracting activity at the same time. That activity could be driving your car, scrolling through Facebook, cooking the dinner, or washing the dishes.

If you can, try to eat at a table, and try to eat your food from a plate. I think that we have all sat down to a cup of tea and eaten biscuits from the packet. If you are interested in eating mindfully, decide how many biscuits you want to eat, take them out of the packet, put them on a plate, and – if possible – sit down at a table to eat them.

Take a moment to notice the food on your plate, become aware of the colours, shape, and smell of the food.

Slowly eat the food, savouring the taste and the smell of it. Permit yourself to enjoy it.

Recognise That You Don't Have to be Perfect

I could write an entire book on self-criticism; it is at the core of so much distress. When we think about making changes to our diets, we need to be realistic and recognise that even small changes are positive and worthwhile. Too many times, people try to make drastic changes to their diet, saying, "I am never going to eat another biscuit" and then when they inevitably eat that biscuit, a familiar story starts to play out in their mind: "I have no willpower," or "I can never stick to a healthy eating plan," or "There is no point," or "I should just give up."

If this sounds familiar to you, see if you can begin to hear that old, habitual story but not take it onboard. What might happen if you heard a new, more compassionate story? "You had a bad day and had some biscuits and a bag of crisps. That's okay, you can eat a healthy lunch," or "Be kind to yourself, you are trying to make changes to your life and you are doing the best you can." If you develop a more compassionate self, you will be able to move forward towards your values with greater ease.

Seek Professional Support

Some people who have significant difficulties with emotional eating may benefit from professional support. Your GP or family doctor should be able to advise you on how to get the help that you need.

Things to Remember

- A poor diet is associated with poor physical *and* mental health.

- Many people can improve their health by drinking more fluids, eating more fruit and vegetables and by reducing their consumption of processed foods and sugar.

- Emotional eating is very common. Most of us do it.

- Reflecting on your reasons for improving your diet can help motivate you to make positive changes to your diet.

- Planning ahead, working with your thoughts, practising mindful eating, and developing a toolbox of self-soothing behaviours can help manage emotional eating.

CHAPTER 13: MAINTAIN GOOD RELATIONSHIPS

> *Relationships are based on four principles: respect, understanding, acceptance, and appreciation.*
>
> ## Mahatma Gandhi

We are all connected to each other. You may be married, you may be in a partnership, you may be single, you may be a member of a big family, you may live alone, but no matter what your circumstances – you are connected to other people. We know that pain does not just affect the person living with it; it also affects the people closest to them.

It is my experience that many people who live with pain try to hide it, at least to some extent, from their friends and family. They tell me things like, "They have enough to cope with in their own lives; I don't want to burden them."

I can understand that you struggle with your pain at times, and you don't want your pain to impact on the people you love, too. However, there is an old saying, "No man is an island" and there is a lot of truth to this statement.

We all live within systems, family systems, networks of friends and communities of people. Just like with any system, when something changes, it inevitably touches upon the other parts of the system. If your car runs out of oil, it will impact on other parts of the engine. Even though you don't want your pain to impact on the systems that you live within, it will undoubtedly have an impact.

Let's think about Sarah. She is very close to her sister, and they often go on holiday and weekend breaks together. When Sarah considers her role within her family, she is aware that she has always been the organiser, and the person who offers solutions to problems. Sarah knows that her sister relies on her a lot – for practical and emotional support. The dynamic between Sarah and her sister is such that Sarah has usually been the one providing the support, rather than requesting it.

Sarah developed significant difficulties with back pain about 18 months ago. Recently, she went away for a long weekend with her sister on a city break. As is usual with many city breaks, Sarah and her sister were determined to do as much sightseeing as possible. This inevitability meant a lot of walking, and on the second day of the break, Sarah noticed that she was finding it difficult to keep up with her sister. She recalled struggling with the many flights of stairs at one of the tourist attractions but felt unable to ask her sister to stop for a break. She didn't feel that she could ask for support, even if that support was just a long coffee break and an earlier return to the hotel. Instead, she fought on and continued walking and climbing the stairs, eventually arriving home at the end of the weekend in total agony.

I spent some time with Sarah exploring why she found it so difficult to be open and honest with her sister about her pain and her need for rest. Sarah admitted that she struggled with the idea of being vulnerable, especially due to her role within the family. I had news for Sarah – she was vulnerable! We are all vulnerable. Sometimes in our lives, we can feel more vulnerable than at other times, but *vulnerability comes with being human.*

Many people struggle with showing their vulnerability and being open and honest about their needs. Some people, like Sarah, have been taught that you should push on and keep a 'stiff upper lip' in times of need. This message was conveyed very powerfully to Sarah in childhood when her father was tragically killed in an accident. In the time following her father's death, Sarah was taught to suppress her emotions, to just get on with it without showing her distress. Sarah had unconsciously adopted it as a blueprint for life.

Let's consider the costs for Sarah in keeping her needs to herself. Does this unwritten rule bring her closer to her values or move her away from them? When she reflected on her situation, Sarah realised that her unwritten rule of rarely communicating her needs didn't serve her. Whatsmore, this rule didn't serve her even *before* she developed her pain. She acknowledged that her life would be better if she let her guard down, if she allowed herself to be vulnerable in the presence of her sister.

Sarah had always loved travelling and experiencing and learning from different cultures. It was important to her that she continued to have these experiences in her life. Sarah realised that to continue to travel regularly, she would need to learn to pace herself and to meet her need for rest. She acknowledged that it was likely that she would always be much more active than normal when she was away on a city break, and she was prepared to experience a temporary increase in her pain. However, she also knew that communicating her needs to her sister would help her enjoy her breaks much more.

Assertive Communication

Some people believe that it is selfish to meet their own needs; that they should always put other people's needs before their own.

Rachel thought like this. She tried to always say yes to people, even though she was sometimes screaming "No!" inside. Deep down, she was afraid that people wouldn't like her unless she always accommodated their requests. As a result, she often ended up doing things that she didn't want to do, and she never prioritised her own needs for rest and relaxation.

From time to time, Rachel 'blew her top', becoming upset and angry. This display of anger felt very uncomfortable to her; she didn't like losing her temper and would very quickly 'put a lid on it' to become her normal, passive self. Rachel realised that her difficulty with being assertive and communicating her needs was problematic for her. She constantly felt exhausted, and often felt used by others. As she said, "I must have 'mug' tattooed on my forehead." She was aware that her difficulty with being assertive impacted on her psychological wellbeing and on her ability to manage her pain and pace her activity.

Rachel decided to do something about her difficulty, and gradually she became more assertive, communicating her needs to her family members and saying "no" to them when she didn't want to do what they asked. How do you think her family members reacted when she started to be more assertive? Do you think that they liked her being assertive? They didn't! They didn't like the fact that she was no longer available to meet their needs as they saw fit, and they found it hard to explain the changes in her that they witnessed. They would say things like, "Rachel is not herself these days. I wonder what is wrong with her?"

As a result of our discussions, Rachel knew to expect some reaction from her family members as they adjusted to her new interactions with them. She also knew that she needed to persevere and that, eventually, her family members would adapt to her new style of communication.

It is very rare to find someone who is consistently passive in their communication, or someone who is assertive all the time, or someone who is always aggressive. However, most people have a communication style that is predominant in their lives, and it is my experience that many individuals have mostly adopted a passive communication style. Because they are not meeting their needs, they also become forceful in their communication from time to time. Like Rachel, such people don't like communicating aggressively and very quickly revert to their usual passive style of communication. Often, their self-esteem is low, and they find that their needs are rarely met.

People also get confused about assertiveness. They assume it is the same as being aggressive. Aggressive people hurt, bully, and intimidate other people, whilst assertive people have the confidence to speak up for themselves, to meet their own needs.

> **If you are assertive, you respect yourself as well as other people. You express thoughts, feelings, and beliefs in direct, honest and appropriate ways. You also respect the thoughts, feelings, and beliefs of others.**

Consider spending a few minutes reflecting on your communication style. Are you usually passive, aggressive, or assertive?

People frequently tell me that they can usually be reasonably assertive with people they don't know very well, but they struggle to be assertive with family and close friends. Is that the case for you?

Other people tell me that they struggle with being assertive across the board – with strangers, acquaintances and family and friends. For example, many people have told me that they would struggle with letting waiting staff in a restaurant know that they were unhappy with their meal, even if, for example, they had paid a lot of money for an expensive steak that was not cooked as requested.

If, upon reflection, you think that you struggle with being assertive, then consider the impact that this has on your psychological wellbeing and your ability to manage your pain. If you decide that you want to start becoming more assertive, there is no time like the present!

Practising assertive communication can be very daunting if you are not used to interacting in this way. Your mind can start to generate a lot of stories, for example, "You are just being selfish by saying no," or "You should *always* be helpful to others," or "People are going to think that all you think about is yourself," and so on and so on.

As with all the stories that our minds generate, it can be helpful to take a step back and consider them a bit more objectively. Does it serve you to always do what other people want? If you meet your own needs, does it mean that you can never help anyone out? Remember that some of the stories our minds generate are helpful to us, but many of them are not.

As with most new skills, when you are learning to become assertive, it can be easier to take 'baby steps' and dip your toe in the assertiveness water. As you become more assertive, your confidence will grow and – like learning any new skill – it will become easier with time and practice.

It is also important to remember that you are likely to be met with some resistance as you become more assertive. Like Rachel in the example above, some of the people around you are unlikely to embrace this change in you with open arms.

As I have referenced several times, people like to maintain the status quo and when someone within our circle or 'system' changes, it forces us to change, and we don't like that.

That's the bad news; the good news is that we all have an amazing capacity to adjust and change – if we didn't, I would be out of a job! Over time, the people in your life will adjust to you being more assertive; they will get used to you communicating clearly to them about your needs, thoughts, and feelings.

Assertive Communication and Pain

As you know, persistent pain changes from day-to-day. It changes in intensity, and for some pain conditions – like Fibromyalgia – the location of the pain may also change. There may be days when you need a lot of practical support, and other days when you may need little, if any, practical support.

> It will be impossible for the people around you to know how much support you need unless you communicate with them. Clear, honest communication is a vital part of living with pain.

When we have been in a relationship for a long time, whether that is a romantic relationship, a sibling relationship, or a parent-child relationship, we often make the mistake of assuming that the other person in the relationship knows what we need.

As we know, there are very few people in this world who have developed mindreading skills! Even if you have been in a relationship with the same person for over twenty years, they will not always know what you are thinking, and they will not be able to respond to your needs unless you communicate clearly.

We all communicate using verbal and non-verbal means. Communication experts tell us that most of our communication is carried out non-verbally. Gestures, body language, facial expressions, and eye contact are all forms of non-verbal communication. It can be difficult to interpret non-verbal communication accurately, and even communication experts struggle with this.

People often tell me that they are reluctant to talk to friends and family about their pain. They might be unwilling to talk about their pain because they don't want to distress their friends and family. Like Sarah in the example above, they may feel uncomfortable showing their vulnerability, or they may view talking about their pain as a pointless exercise because they believe that there is nothing anyone can do to help them. However, we know that even if people who live with pain do not *talk* about their pain verbally, their pain and distress will undoubtedly be communicated *non-verbally*.

I can remember slipping heavily on ice one winter morning on my way to work. I really hurt my tail bone, but I had to get to work – I was running a group for people with pain that morning. I had no way of contacting the group members as I was travelling directly from home, and I didn't want them to turn up to the session and for me not to be there.

Living out my (unhelpful) rule that you should not miss work, even if you are not well, I drove to the group, in agony. I walked into the room, intending to hide my pain and act like a professional. The moment I walked into the room, some concerned patients asked me what was wrong and a few of them said, "I can see the pain on your face." I was shocked at how quickly I had been rumbled and how easily my pain had 'leaked out' into my facial expression.

I am not suggesting that you talk about your pain, non-stop, all day, every day. That wouldn't be helpful for you or your family and friends. But it is helpful to have conversations about your pain, how it impacts on you, and how other people can support you.

The support may involve practical help, "I am going to drive for the first half-hour of the journey and then I am going to stop for a few minutes to stretch my legs. Could you drive the last half hour of the journey?" or "I am going to try to go for a 15-minute walk three times a week. I would love it if you helped motivate me to do it by walking with me." At times, you may require emotional support, "I am feeling down today. Could you sit and have a cup of tea and a chat with me?"

It is important to remember that, very often, your friends and family members also feel frustrated by your pain and your suffering. It can be hard for them to understand why your pain is persisting, and why there has not been a medical cure for it. Don't forget that everyone – including your friends and family members – has experienced pain, but for the majority of them, that pain has been short-lasting acute pain.

As this is their experience of pain, is it any wonder that they struggle to understand the persistent nature of your pain and the fact that it does not appear to have been 'cured' by the medication that your doctor has prescribed? In an attempt to help them understand living with persistent pain a little better, you could suggest that close family members or friends read some, or all, of this book. At the very least, it would be helpful if they read the first chapter on understanding the nature of persistent pain.

It would also be helpful if your family members and friends understand that it is beneficial to become more active when you live with pain. If they understand a little bit about the pacing of activity, they will be able to support you with pacing and will not become confused when you don't complete a task immediately; for example, when you only mow one side of the lawn.

I regularly meet with the family members of people who are living with pain, and they consistently express the desire to support their loved ones. They frequently say that it is helpful when their family member lets them know how they can assist them.

Friends or family members can be a great support when you are working on pain management goals. For example, if you are trying to become more active, they could encourage you to go for that walk or swim, or they could get active with you. If you want to begin to practise meditation regularly, they could give you the ten minutes of uninterrupted time that you need to practise. They could help you (and themselves) with sleep by skipping that evening coffee.

> **Friends and family members won't be able to encourage you if you don't have a conversation about your pain and what you are hoping to change in your life.**

At the beginning of this book, I outlined some of the ways that living with persistent pain can impact on the people experiencing it. Many patients have told me that they have experienced a loss of independence and a lowering of their self-esteem since they developed their pain. People who live with pain may need help with certain self-care tasks; for example, putting on socks and shoes. People may need help lifting heavy saucepans; they may need help cutting down the bushes in the garden. Sometimes family members inadvertently add to the distress of the person living with pain by doing more and more for them, which reduces their independence, leading further to lower self-esteem and impacting negatively on their psychological wellbeing.

I can recall Bob's story of his children and grandchildren visiting. Bob told me that his family came to visit him every Sunday and that he loved to see them coming. It was a tradition in his family to put on the kettle as soon as visitors arrived. Bob told me that when his adult children arrived to visit him on a Sunday, they refused to let him get up from the sofa, insisting that they made the tea. Bob was distressed by this; he was very capable of making tea and sandwiches for his family and wanted to do it. In an attempt to show their care and love for him, Bob's family had taken this 'job' away from him. This made Bob feel even worse about himself, "I can't even make a cup of tea for them now."

After we had discussed this situation, Bob agreed to talk to his family about his feelings. When he broached the subject initially, his children did their usual thing of telling him it was fine, that they didn't mind making the tea. Instead of dropping the subject, Bob took time to let them know that it was really important to him to make tea and sandwiches for them, and that this form of hosting made him feel good. As a result of this conversation, Bob's children became aware of the importance of Bob maintaining his independence by showing his love and care for his children by making them tea.

Ryan was married with three teenage children. He noticed that he had become more irritable since he developed his pain. He described himself as an 'easy-going person' before he developed his pain, but now the smallest thing seemed to annoy him. He often 'bit the head off' his wife and children, and he felt guilty and upset after he had lashed out at them.

Ryan had become increasingly withdrawn since he developed his pain. He rarely went out with friends anymore, and even when he was at home with his family, he noticed that he had become very withdrawn, often going to another room or going to bed early, just to be on his own.

Ryan's wife, Jane, was worried about him. She hated to see him in pain, but she didn't know how to help him. She was afraid to bring up the subject of his pain in case it caused an argument or made him feel worse.

While it was undoubtedly difficult for Ryan and Jane to begin to have a conversation about his pain, and the impact that it had on their relationship, it was helpful for them to open up to each other. Ryan let Jane know how difficult it was for him to live with his pain, plus the things she said and did that helped him cope, and the things she said and did that were not helpful for him.

Jane talked to Ryan about how difficult it was for her to see him in pain. She told him that she noticed how withdrawn he had become and that it was important for her to spend time with him and to reconnect. Ryan and Jane were both upset during this conversation, but they were glad that they had talked and they believed that they would be able to move forward together.

Persistent Pain and Sexual Relationships

All couples go through phases when they don't have time or the energy for sex. For many couples, medical and psychological issues also cause difficulties in their sexual relationship.

It is very common for pain to impact on sexual relationships. Many patients have told me that they have become much less

214

physically intimate since they developed their pain. They may be fearful of hurting themselves or causing even more pain, or their partner may be reluctant to be physically intimate as they are concerned about hurting the person living with pain.

When you live with pain, your libido – or sexual desire – may be affected. You might remember from a previous chapter that low libido is one of the symptoms of depression and if you are living with pain and are also depressed, it is more likely that your libido will be low. Many people tell me that their body confidence has become much lower since they developed pain, and we know that this can also impact on sexual relationships. It is very common to put on weight when you are living with pain, and many people tell me that they feel self-conscious about their weight gain. Some individuals tell me that they are no longer comfortable being naked in the presence of their partner because of their weight gain and lack of body confidence.

Anna had been married for nine years and had two young daughters, aged ten and eight. Before she developed her back pain, she was living a very active life, working part-time and caring for her children. She went to boxercise twice a week with two of her friends. She enjoyed the workout and the chat after the class.

Anna had to give up her work two years ago because of her pain. Before she developed her pain, she loved cooking and baking. Since developing her pain, she struggled to lift heavy saucepans and she had lost her interest in baking. She used to meet her friends for a girl's night out once a month. She rarely went out with them now; she was usually too tired and sore in the evenings to make the effort to meet them.

Before she developed her pain, Anna used to go out with her husband for dinner every couple of weeks. She had only been out for dinner with him a few times since she developed her pain. Anna stopped going to boxercise about three years ago and didn't do any exercise anymore. Anna usually went to bed shortly after her daughters. She watched TV in bed for an hour or two before going to sleep while her husband watched TV in the sitting room. She felt guilty that her husband was left sitting alone downstairs, but she was so exhausted by her pain that she just wanted to lie down.

Anna felt guilty about the impact that her pain had on her family. Her husband worked long hours and had to come home in the evening and help her with some of the housework and help her with the evening meal. She knew that he enjoyed going out for dinner, and she felt bad that she didn't have the energy to do that anymore.

Anna had not had sex with her husband in over a year. She didn't seem to have an interest in sex anymore. Anna had put on weight, over two stone, in the past two years. She was upset by her weight gain and worried that her husband did not find her attractive anymore.

Anna was worried about her relationship with her husband. She was worried that he would get fed up and leave her, or that he would meet somebody else. Anna knew that she would be devastated if her husband left her. She loved him and couldn't imagine life without him. Anna knew that she should talk to her husband about how she was feeling, but she was too scared to broach the subject in case he told her that he no longer wanted to be in a relationship with her. Anna kept her worries to herself, but she wished that things could be different.

Jamie was Anna's husband. He was worried about her. She hardly ever saw her friends and she never seemed to want to go out anymore. He suspected that she was depressed, but he didn't know what to do to help her. He knew that her back was sore and he didn't mind helping out with the housework or the dinner in the evenings. Jamie had noticed that there was very little physical intimacy between him and Anna anymore. If he tried to hug her, she quickly pulled away. He wondered if she didn't find him attractive anymore. Jamie wanted to be more intimate with Anna again; he just doesn't know what to do.

Using Anna's life as an example, take a moment to imagine some of the stories that were likely to be playing out for her. It was likely that she frequently got caught up or *fused* with stories about being a 'bad wife', about being 'a burden'. Her mind was likely to conjure very frightening stories about how her marriage could not go on like this, about how Jamie was going to look for someone else, someone who was able to be a 'proper wife' to him.

Also, consider some of the reasons why Anna might have pulled away from Jamie when he tried to hug her. In Anna's mind, a story was being played out about how it would be unfair to respond to Jamie's hugs as that would just be 'leading him on' when she was too tired to become more intimate with him.

If you were friends with Anna and Jamie, and they asked you for advice, what would you say? I guess the first thing that you would suggest is to talk.

Sex is a very intimate, personal issue, and many people find it embarrassing to talk about. However, we know that communication is a core part of overcoming any relationship difficulties, including sexual ones. You can see from Anna and Jamie's story that they were both worried about their relationship. Anna was worried that Jamie would get fed up and leave her for someone else. Jamie was worried that Anna didn't find him attractive anymore. We can also see that physical intimacy was important for both Anna and Jamie, and they both wanted this area of their relationship to improve.

While some couples are happy to live a contented life without having a sexual relationship, many couples that I see want to improve this aspect of their lives together. I have listed several tips to consider below.

Tips for Working on your Sexual Relationship

Talk to your Partner

As I wrote a moment ago, this may feel embarrassing or difficult, especially if you have not spoken about sex in a long time. Some people may never have had a conversation about sex with their partner before. It is best to have this conversation when you are both relaxed and have the privacy needed to have a good chat. It can also be helpful to state what you notice about your sexual relationship, for example, "I notice that we don't have sex very often anymore," rather than criticising your partner.

Many people have told me that they one of the reasons they avoid talking about their sexual relationship is because they are fearful of what they might hear, and as a result, sex becomes the 'elephant in the room'. If you start a conversation about sex, it is important that you express your thoughts and views but that your partner is also allowed the time to express his/her thoughts and views too. While you may feel anxious about hearing what your partner thinks and feels, it is important to have an open and honest conversation so that you can find a way to move forward.

It is also helpful to remember that everyone is different when it comes to their sexual relationships and how they would like them to be. I can recall one woman telling me that she was distressed because her sexual relationship had changed since she developed her pain, and that she was having sex much less frequently now, about once a year. A couple of weeks later, another woman told me that her sexual relationship had also deteriorated and that she was having sex much less frequently as well, only about three times a week. This, too, was distressing for her.

Many things influence how we think about sexual relationships, including our relationship history, our culture, and the way sex was perceived and talked about when we were growing up in our family of origin. It is important to remember that your partner may have a different perspective on what he/she would like their sexual relationship to be like. This does not mean that they are right and you are wrong in how you think about it; it also doesn't mean that you are right and they are wrong. Different perspectives just highlight the need for communication.

Gradually Work Your Way Towards Becoming More Physically Intimate

As I said previously, it is very common for people to tell me that they have not been sexually intimate in a long time, sometimes months and years. Sex can seem like a daunting prospect. I can recall one woman telling me that it felt like she had to start again and have sex with her husband for the first time, even though she was happily married and had an active sex life with her husband before the development of her pain.

When sex is a daunting prospect, it becomes very easy to do what people tend to do when faced with daunting issues – avoid it altogether. Many people tell me that they have now become avoidant of physical intimacy most of the time as they are concerned that if they do reach out and hold their partner's hand, or if they do return that lingering kiss, one thing will lead to another, and they will end up having sex – something that is anxiety-provoking for them.

One way of overcoming this difficulty is to develop a plan to become more physically intimate by taking sex off the agenda completely. As I wrote above, we know that a lot of anxiety can come from fears that physical intimacy and any kind of sensual touch can lead to 'full sex'. If you are concerned that you are not going to be able to 'perform', for whatever reason, you are going to avoid intimacy. Applying a ban on sex, even temporarily, can help remove this anxiety and free you up to begin to enjoy physical intimacy and sensual touch again.

> **You and your partner might want to consider ways that you can gradually begin to re-introduce more physical intimacy into your relationship.**

You can work out a pace that is comfortable for both of you. Depending on your current levels of intimacy, this may involve sitting in the same room in the evening to watch TV, it may mean holding hands more often, it may mean kissing more frequently. You may want to try massage as a way of becoming more intimate. One woman told me that she decided to work on getting dressed and undressed in front of her partner again. Her body image had been negatively affected by her pain and she had been dressing and undressing in the bathroom as she was worried that if her husband saw her naked, he would be disgusted by the weight she had put on since she developed her pain.

Once you have begun to become more physically intimate, you may decide to move onto other sexual acts such as intimate touching. You can both decide to leave full sex off the menu until you decide that you are ready. It has been my experience that for many people, full sex happens spontaneously when the couple have reduced the pressure that they have placed on themselves.

It is important to remember that you can be sexually intimate with your partner without having full intercourse. Depending on your circumstances, you and your partner may decide that full intercourse is not something that you want to happen. Couples can have a satisfying sex life without having full intercourse.

If you want to work on improving your sex life, it can helpful if you 'practise' often. People sometimes say that they experience arousal difficulties due to lack of practise – sex is no longer part of their lives. They often find that when they practise being more intimate with their partner, their ability to become aroused improves. However, it is important to remember that it is helpful for people to 'practise' in a relaxed environment where the pressure to perform is removed.

It may be necessary to experiment with positions, depending on the location of your pain. Your 'old' positions may no longer be comfortable for you now that you are living with pain. Like physical exercise and increasing activity levels, sex in a loving relationship will not harm you or damage your body. However, if you have intercourse for the first time in a while, you may notice a temporary increase in your pain. It is important to remember that if you do notice an increase in your pain, it is just temporary and does not indicate that you have damaged yourself.

Pace Yourself

I have talked quite a bit about the pacing of activity, and when we think about sex, it can be helpful to think about pacing it in the same way that you would pace any physical activity. Traditionally, most people have sex at night before they go to sleep. However, if you live with pain, this may be the time of day when you are most sore and tired. It can be helpful to think about the timing of intimacy. I can recall having this conversation with one couple. The woman in the relationship lived with pain. She had not been physically intimate with her partner for some time and was keen to work on this with him. They had always been intimate at night in bed. However, she noticed her pain was worse in the evening, and all she wanted to do at night was roll into bed and try to get some sleep.

We talked about the timing of intimacy and both of them agreed that it would be worth considering being intimate earlier in the day when she was not as sore. Her partner worked shifts and they had no children, so this option would potentially work for them. They agreed to try this, but the woman voiced her concern about what the neighbours would think! We laughed about this and agreed that there was no need to advertise her intentions to her neighbours, and that it didn't matter if they noticed that her curtains were closed for a while during the day.

A Sense of Humour Goes a Long Way

I am a great believer in the benefits of laughter. Many people have told me that using laughter and a sense of humour has helped them when they have been working on improving their sexual relationship with their partner.

Don't Be Afraid to Seek Professional Help

If you think these tips are not enough to help your situation, please consider getting professional help. Your GP or doctor may be able to help, or they may be able to refer you to a specialist colleague or service. Please do not be embarrassed about seeking help. Sexual difficulties are common, and there is help available – there is no need to suffer in silence.

You may be experiencing physical difficulties that are impacting on your sexual relationship. Some pain medications can affect sexual functioning, too. For example, opioid medication can lower testosterone levels, suppressing sexual function in men and causing erectile dysfunction. Medication can also contribute to difficulties with low libido and difficulty with orgasm in both sexes. If you believe that you are experiencing such difficulties, which are impacting on your sexual relationship, it is worth talking this over with your GP or doctor.

Some couples experience sexual difficulties as a result of relationship difficulties. If you think this is the case for you, it is worth considering going for relationship counselling. Your GP or doctor should be able to offer advice on how to access this. Alternatively, you could research professional relationship counselling services in your local area; many of these organisations accept self-referrals.

Things to Remember

- Pain does not just affect the person living with pain; it also affects the people closest to them.

- It can be helpful to spend some time reflecting on your communication style. It is important to be assertive in your communication.

- When you live with pain, you often communicate your pain non-verbally. This type of communication can be hard to interpret. It can be helpful to communicate your thoughts and feelings verbally in an honest, clear, and direct way.

- It is common for pain to impact on sexual relationships.

- There are strategies that can help to improve sexual relationships.

CHAPTER 14: PUTTING IT ALL TOGETHER

> Grant me the serenity to accept the things that I cannot, the courage to change the things that I can, and the wisdom to know the difference.

We all struggle against pain, be it emotional or physical pain. Unfortunately, a lot of the suffering that we experience is a result of our constant struggle against pain. When we feel doubt, fear, anxiety, anger, and physical pain, we struggle against it and try to get rid of it by blocking it out, numbing it out or – as is often the case with persistent pain – making our lives smaller and smaller in an attempt to avoid these unwanted experiences.

The alternative to the struggle to avoid pain is acceptance. Acceptance is a difficult concept to get your head around; many people believe that acceptance means that you have to like (or want) your situation. Who in their right mind would want to live with persistent pain if they were given a choice?

> The origin of the word acceptance can be traced back to a Latin word meaning 'to take or receive what is offered'.

In my mind, acceptance is about taking what you have been given in life, and living a valued life with all that you have been given – even if you have been given a back that causes you pain, or a condition like Fibromyalgia that is associated with widespread pain and fatigue.

When I discuss the concept of acceptance with people, they often become tearful and upset. Most people who live with persistent pain know it is likely that they will have to live with some level of pain, but they struggle to accept it and *allow* this pain to be part of their lives. But what is the alternative – living a 'half-life', where you are alive and breathing, but not really living? Struggling against the pain so much that you no longer do many of the things that bring meaning to your life?

When I talk about acceptance, I often use a metaphor of quicksand that was first described by the Psychologist Dr Steven Hayes. I want you to imagine that you are walking along a beach on a beautiful sunny day. You know exactly where you are going on your walk and how long it will take you to get there. You have planned what you want to do with the rest of your day after you have finished your walk. As you are walking along, you fail to notice some quicksand. You step into it and quickly begin to sink. Your mind is screaming at you, "Get out quickly or you are going to die." In your panic and struggle, you sink faster and faster.

You realise that the harder you are struggling to get out of the quicksand, the faster you are sinking. You accept that you are stuck in the quicksand and that fighting it is making your situation worse. Your fight is not helping you move towards where you want to be. You know that while you did not plan to walk into the quicksand, it is where you are now and what you need to do is give up the struggle, spread out your body weight, and take slow, deliberate movements towards where you want to be.

> **The quicksand principle can be applied to emotional distress and physical pain.**

If you can learn to sit with difficult thoughts, emotions, and physical pain, you will find that the life you live is fuller and more meaningful than a life of struggle where you fight to rid yourself of your distress.

The human instinct to avoid and control distress is so strong that you may not even be aware that you are doing it. It is worth taking some time out to think about *what* you do to avoid distress, be it emotional or physical distress.

Consider the questions below.

- Do you miss out on going to important activities and events due to a desire to control your pain, or your anxiety, or some other distressing experience?

- Do you engage in activities that help you numb out or escape difficult emotional or physical experiences – like spending hours online or drinking too much?

- Have you done more or less with your life since you developed persistent pain?

Take a moment to think about all the things you do to help manage distressing thoughts, emotions, and physical pain.

- Are these things working for you, or is there another way? If these strategies work for you, do they only work in the short-term? What about their effectiveness in the long-term?

- Are there areas in your life that are worth the experience of pain? If so, what are these areas?

Now would be a good time to review the work that you carried out on values in Chapter 2. Spend some time reflecting. Reflect on what is important to you in your life; what gives your life meaning. Are you moving towards your values and living a fulfilled life? Or are you moving away from the life that you want in an attempt to control your emotional and/or physical distress?

For most people, learning to accept a chronic health condition isn't easy. Although we may never sit down and formally plan our future lives, most of us have a fairly good idea about how we want to live our lives. We might know whether we want to have a family, a particular kind of job or career, and where we want to live.

When you develop persistent pain, it often feels like your roadmap for your future has been taken away and ripped up. A new, more unclear roadmap has been presented to you, and it can take a lot of time to get your head around it. You may constantly think about how unfair your situation is, and long for your old life – that familiar roadmap. Unfortunately, if you put all your energy into fighting and trying to escape from your situation, and if you don't adapt to this new life and your new reality, it is likely that your quality of life will significantly deteriorate.

When we consider the concept of acceptance, it can be helpful to think of the serenity appeal, part of which is quoted at the very beginning of this chapter. No matter how much we dislike them, there are some aspects of our lives that we cannot change. They cannot be changed no matter how much energy we put into changing them. I have known some people who have wasted *years of their lives* trying to transform aspects of their life that they will never be able to change. While they are putting all their energy into trying to change the impossible, they have been blinded to what they could do to improve their lives.

The second part of the serenity appeal refers to just that, the things in life that we can change to allow us to live a more meaningful, fulfilled life. Setting goals can help us make positive changes in our lives, and I will discuss setting goals in more detail later in this chapter.

Finally, the last part of the serenity appeal talks about having the wisdom to know what parts of life you need to accept and what parts of life you can change. That can be tricky to figure out. It may be hard to admit that there are aspects of life that you need to accept, and it can be hard to find the courage and motivation to change the aspects of your life that you can change.

Acceptance of your situation involves making adaptations and alterations to your life. It often means setting goals in various areas so that you can live a full life again. Reflecting on your values can help you set those goals. Your life may never be the same as it is was before you developed persistent pain, but that doesn't mean that you can't have a full, happy, and successful life. This is still achievable, even if your pain persists.

Setting Goals

Now that you are coming close to the end of this book, take the time to set goals that will help you move toward your values, and closer to the life that is important to you. The people reading this book will all live different lives and have different needs; some may want to focus on their sleep, others may want to focus on improving their relationships, some will want to start a regular mindfulness meditation practice. Many people may wish to work on overcoming their fears about activity and exercise by gradually increasing their activity levels. Choose to set goals in different areas of life.

The following exercise is well worth attempting. Take out a notebook or a piece of paper and write down today's date. Then cross out the year on the date and change it to next year. Now you have the date for this time next year.

What do you want your life to look like this time next year? Do you want it to be better or worse? The choices that you make today, and over the next year, will determine what your life looks like on the date that you have written down. You have choices to make.

Let's use a crossroads on a country road as a metaphor. You have five choices when you stand at that crossroads. You can go straight ahead, turn left, or turn right. You can do a U-turn and go back the way you came. Or you can stand at the crossroads and let life whizz past you. Only you can decide which way to go.

It can be frightening standing at the crossroads as you are not sure where the roads will lead you. You may not believe that you have the energy or the motivation to move from the crossroads. However, I believe that if you have picked up this book and have read this far, you want to make changes and travel down new roads. I believe that the fact you are reading these words indicates you are not content to stand at the crossroads… watching life whizz by.

Types of Goals

When we think about goals, it is helpful to think about short-, medium-, and long-term goals. Your long-term goal may be something that you want to achieve in the next six months, next year, or within the next two years. Your medium-term goal may be what you want to achieve in the next month. Your short-term goal might be what you want to achieve today.

Writing goals down makes it more likely that you will achieve them.

I encourage the people that I work with to write down their goals and to read them frequently. If you are struggling with your motivation, it is helpful to spend some time before bed in the evening, or first thing in the morning, writing down your goals for the day.

Many people who live with persistent pain have told me that their life has become like Groundhog Day – every day seems the same. Writing a daily list of goals can help break into the Groundhog Day cycle. Actually, it is good to set goals in life, whether you live with persistent pain or not. It is easy to drift through life not thinking about what you want to do, or how you want to live your life. But life is short – think how quickly a year passes by. It is a cliché but still worth saying, we only have one life and we can all live a good one – even if life has thrown a curveball at us.

> # Traditionally, when we consider goal setting, we talk about setting SMART goals.

I will break SMART goals down for you.

S > Specific Goals

This means being very specific about what you want to achieve. For example, I might set myself the goal of 'being more active'. That goal is vague; what does 'being more active' really mean? However, if I set the goal of 'walking for 15 minutes, 3 times a week', it is very specific. At the end of the week, I can easily recognise whether I have met my goal or not.

M > Measurable Goals

Sometimes, when we set ourselves goals, it is hard to tell if we have achieved them or not. If we set measurable goals, we will be able to know if and when we have achieved them. A patient that I worked with, recently, told me that he wanted to spend some more time with his partner as he felt that their relationship had deteriorated since he developed his pain. He set himself the measurable goal of spending *half an hour with his partner every evening after work*, when they would spend time chatting about their day without the distraction of a TV or a phone. This goal is measurable and he could easily tell if he had achieved it.

A > Achievable Goals

It has been my experience that this aspect of goal setting is most challenging for people who live with persistent pain. People who live with pain often set the bar for their goal too high. Why? Because they are basing their goal on their *former* pre-pain self. This is very apparent, especially when it comes to activity and exercise goals.

I am going to use the example of Jacqui, who ran marathons in the past (indeed, I think that she ran about nine or ten in total). When Jacqui developed persistent back and leg pain, she gave up her running, which was devastating for her. In the few years after she developed her pain, she became more and more inactive. When she came to see me, she wanted to work on improving her exercise tolerance and physical fitness. She had become depressed, and she (rightly) thought that regular exercise might improve her mood and help her manage her pain.

Jacqui struggled with setting achievable activity goals. Given her baseline activity level, we agreed that it was achievable for her to set an initial goal of walking for 20 minutes, three times a week. Even though Jacqui understood that it was an achievable initial goal for her, her mind had plenty to say about that goal! "That is pathetic, seriously a 20-minute walk!" and "What good is a 20-minute walk going to do you?" and "You have gone from running marathons to a 20-minute walk at a snail's pace – is that the best that you can do?"

Jacqui had some choices to make. One of her options was to listen to her mind and give up on her goal of becoming more active. Or she could push herself way beyond her achievable goal and walk for longer, perhaps walking for 40 minutes to an hour.

Let's look at the potential outcomes of those different options. If Jacqui gives up on her exercise goal, she is likely to become even more deconditioned, which would not be good for her mental or physical health. If she decides to push forward beyond her achievable goal, she will likely be able to manage a few days of it at most, before it becomes too much. She would likely enter that boom or bust cycle that I talked about earlier in the book. She is then likely to feel even worse about herself and her situation.

The third option for Jacqui is to hear what her mind has to say about her 20-minute walking goal, to become aware of what the passengers on her bus have to say. She can then choose to do her own thing – 'drive her own bus' – and move towards her values by working on the achievable goal that she has set herself.

Jacqui will likely be able to walk for an hour, three times a week in the future, but right now, this goal is not achievable. Given her baseline, a 20-minute walk, three times a week, is a good short-term goal for her. When her exercise tolerance and her confidence increase, she can set a new goal, gradually working her way towards her long-term activity goal.

R > Relevant Goals

When you think about setting goals, it is important to set goals that are relevant to your life. What would make your life more meaningful? What would move you towards your values? When I am working with people, *I* don't decide what goals they should work on. The person themself decides what areas of life they want to focus on, and what goals they want to set within that area of life.

Sometimes, people struggle to come up with goals. They don't know where to begin. If you have carried out the values work in Chapter 2, you could reflect on this work to help you decide on your goals.

Are there one or two areas of your life where you feel that you are *not* successfully living out your values? When you read through the various chapters of this book, did some jump out at you more than others? These may be the areas that you want to work on.

T > Time-Based

Setting goals that are time-based can help us obtain a sense of achievement. For many people living with persistent pain, their mind is full of chatter about how useless they are, and how little they achieve on a daily, weekly, and monthly basis. As I have mentioned before, people consistently tell me that their self-confidence and self-esteem has become significantly lower since they developed their pain. Setting and achieving goals helps their self-confidence and self-esteem improve.

However, I need to give you a word of warning here. Let's go back to Jacqui's goal regarding her activity levels. Imagine that Jacqui managed to work with her mental chatter and set herself the goal of 20 minutes walking, three times a week. This goal is time-based, and she has set herself the goal of achieving it within a week.

What would happen if Jacqui got a tummy bug and didn't get the opportunity to walk on three occasions? What if Jacqui's mind started to chatter about her 'failure' to achieve her goal only one week into starting to work on them? What if her mind told her to give up her goal of walking by telling her that there was no point in even trying (as life would always get in the way)? I know that if Jacqui took her mind's chatter on board, it would be much more likely that she would give up on her goal. If Jacqui managed to become an observer of her thoughts – without being pulled into the stories of her mind – she could persist with her walking goal and continue to move towards her values.

Life is unpredictable. Persistent pain can be unpredictable. There may be days when you feel that your life is going down a predictable path, and there may be days when you feel you have little control over your life. It will be necessary to adjust your goals from time to time due to this unpredictability.

For example, you may have decided to set a goal to achieve something within a month, but – due to changing circumstances – you may have to adjust that time frame to six weeks or two months. It is important that you become aware of your mind's chatter around this; if you become aware that your mind has become very critical, try observing this critical chatter, rather than becoming fused with it and hooking onto the stories in your mind. Choose not to take that criticism on board!

> **If you don't become fused with your critical and unhelpful thoughts, you are much more likely to be able to move forward with your goals.**

It is really important to remember that when you are working on your goals, you *will have* ups and downs – good days and bad days. It is very rare to achieve a goal without any challenges or difficulties.

Earlier in this book, I asked you to think about something that you have achieved in life, and whether it was easy to achieve. I will ask you to consider this question again. So often, we set goals and give up when we face a challenge. We assume that we can't do it, that it is too hard, that it wasn't meant for us.

Perseverance is the key to achieving goals.

You may have to modify your goal, you may have to add a few more steps to help you get there, but if you persevere and believe in your capabilities, you will be able to achieve far more than you ever dreamed was possible.

Self-Compassion

When I think about goal setting, I have to mention self-compassion – or the lack of it(!) – that I observe so often in the people that I work with. It is my experience that many people, especially those who live with pain, struggle to be compassionate towards themselves.

What is Compassion?

One definition of compassion that is often used by psychologists was offered by The Dalai Lama, who described it as "a sensitivity to the suffering in the self and others, with a commitment to try to alleviate and prevent it." I find that many people who live with pain are compassionate towards other people but struggle to show themselves any compassion. Instead of being sensitive to their suffering, they are frequently self-critical, often engaging in toxic self-talk.

When we look at the definition of compassion that I used above, we can see two parts to the definition. The first part involves a sensitivity to suffering.

> **It is important to remember that you did not choose to live a life in pain, and that you are doing the best you can.**

The second part of the definition involves the commitment to try to alleviate and prevent it. This implies that you have a responsibility to relieve your suffering, to do the things that you know will make your life better.

When I discuss compassion with people, especially showing compassion to the self, they often declare that such behaviour might be interpreted as a sign of weakness or self-indulgence. However, we know that compassion is not weak or self-indulgent at all.

Think of someone you know, either in your own life or someone well-known on the world stage, who you would regard as compassionate. Do you believe that this person is weak or indulgent? I would say not. Then why is it weak or self-indulgent to be compassionate towards yourself?

> **It takes strength and courage to turn inwards and look at your distress and suffering. It also takes dedication and wisdom to take action to alleviate the suffering.**

When you notice that your mind is being critical or judgemental, or when you notice that your mind is telling you scary stories about your situation, it is helpful to imagine what your compassionate self might say. This can be difficult at first; many people are not used to being compassionate towards themselves. Let's use the example of Jacqui's situation from earlier in this chapter.

What would Jacqui's compassionate self say about her situation? It might say something like this, "Jacqui, you have been through a really difficult couple of years. Life has been hard, and you have had to adjust to massive changes. You have felt great sadness about the fact that you gave up your running; you loved doing marathons. You have tried to cope with your pain and the changes in your life as well as you could. You are trying to move forward with your life, and you are committed to doing everything that you can to improve your life. You made a great start by walking twice last week. You did the best you could. Now that tummy bug has cleared up, you can start to do your walking again."

Affirmations

I want to finish the book by talking to you about the power of positive affirmations.

> **Positive affirmations are positive statements made about the self that you repeat frequently, at least daily if possible.**

Examples of affirmations include, "I am kind to myself," and "I am brave." Affirmations work best if you repeat them often. To remember to do this, you can 'anchor' your affirmations to something that you do routinely; for example, when you brush your teeth, or when you boil the kettle to make a cup of tea.

It can be helpful to have your affirmations written down somewhere you can easily access them, perhaps stuck in a visible place in your bedroom or on the notes page of your phone.

You can consider trying out different affirmations that resonate with you and where you are in your life. You can change these affirmations depending on what is going on in your life.

Try saying the affirmations out loud if you are alone. You may feel a bit silly doing this at first, but try to persevere. You can also say the affirmations silently in your mind.

When you are repeating the affirmation, try to imagine yourself being that person. For example, if your affirmation is "I am confident," you can imagine yourself as that confident person when you repeat your affirmation. What would you look like if you were that person, how would you act, how would people respond to you?

> ## Affirmations can be helpful when you repeat them often and when you believe in them.

The last part of this statement is important. For affirmations to be effective, you must be able to believe them, at least to some extent. I want you to imagine that you had a really poor body image. You truly thought that your body was disgusting. What would happen if you pasted the positive affirmation "My body is beautiful" on your mirror and began to recite it regularly? Your mind would very quickly jump in and list numerous reasons why this is not the case and why you are far from beautiful. At best, this affirmation will do nothing at all to help your body image, and at worst, it will make it even worse. We can't talk ourselves into something that we just don't believe.

A better approach is to bring awareness to our thoughts and notice what our mind is telling us. Then we can re-frame our thoughts by coming up with an affirmation, or positive self-statement, that we do believe, at least to some extent.

For example, consider Annie, whose mind frequently tells her that she is not a good enough mother because she cannot be as active with her children as she would like. When Annie reflected on her relationship with her adolescent daughter, Ellen, she realised that Ellen has a very open relationship with her and seems able to talk to her about any worries or difficulties that she is experiencing in her life. Several of Annie's friends have commented on this, saying that they envy the close relationship that Annie has with her daughter. Annie could come up with the positive affirmation, "I can give Ellen the emotional support that she needs." This is a good affirmation for Annie as it is positively framed and is credible to her. In contrast, "I am not a bad mother" is not a good affirmation as it is framed negatively.

You might consider devising a few affirmations or 'I statements', remembering that it is important to frame them positively. If you are struggling to develop any believable positive affirmations, you could say something like, "I am working on the belief that I am good at my job" or "I am working on the belief that it is safe for me to become more active." These affirmations can help you change your mindset and overcome the limiting beliefs that you undoubtedly have. I have used the phrase "undoubtedly have" because everyone has some limiting beliefs.

If you are trying to become more active, it might be helpful for you to have some positive affirmations that you can use at the time or when you are exercising. You might consider repeating statements like "My body is getting stronger" or "I am getting fitter and healthier" when you are exercising or even when you are carrying out household tasks. I know that when I am lifting weights at the gym – something I don't have a natural talent for – I tell myself, "my body is strong and healthy." This seems to help maintain a more positive attitude in the gym and helps me turn down the volume on my mind when it says that I am not as strong as the other women in the class and that I may as well go home.

What we think, say, and believe about ourselves becomes our reality. If we believe that we cannot do something, we won't even try. A powerful example of this is the four-minute mile. Scientists used to believe that nobody could run a mile in less than four minutes. They believed that the human body was literally incapable of such a feat, and over the years, many people tried and failed to do it, proving the scientists right.

In 1954, Roger Bannister ran a mile in three minutes and 59.4 seconds. What do you think happened in the years following Mr Bannister's achievement? Since 1954, more than 1,500 runners have also achieved the impossible and run a mile in under four minutes. How do you think that this happened? Did the human body suddenly evolve into something capable of running a mile in less than four minutes? Or was it that people's beliefs about their potential capabilities changed? The runners' mindsets transformed, and they managed to do the 'impossible' because they believed they could do it.

I want to ask you a question? Do you believe you have reached your full potential in every area of your life? No one I have ever asked has answered "Yes". When I ask myself the same question, I have to say that I don't believe I have achieved my full potential in every area of my life.

What holds us back from reaching our potential? Just like the runners before 1954 who tried to run a mile in under four minutes, our *limiting beliefs* hold us back. That chatter in our mind, that we become so fused to, dictates so much of our life. This chatter that tells us not to step outside our comfort zone; this chatter that tells us we are not good enough, smart enough, or healthy enough to achieve our goals. What if our minds are wrong? What if we could listen to the doubting, negative chatter but choose to ignore it and move towards our values with courage and determination? How could your life change? How could your life be better? How could your life be more meaningful?

We all have the potential to change, to re-wire our brains. After all, my profession is based on the capacity to change, to make our lives better.

> **No matter what your life is like, no matter how poor your physical or your mental health, you *can* improve it.**

You may be able to bring about change on your own or with the help of family and friends, or you may need professional support to help you with these advancements, but you definitely *can* make them.

I have worked with many people who are living a life with pain who have taken many courageous steps towards a better life. As they took their often-challenging steps, their minds weren't silent; their minds warned them, their minds doubted, and their minds criticised. But these people chose to move forward, through the ups and downs of life, with courage and conviction. Whatever your circumstances, I know that you can do this too. I firmly believe that you can have a life of meaning, even if you are in pain, and I really hope that you have found some hope and encouragement in the pages of this book.

> *Promise me you'll always remember: you're braver than you believe, stronger than you seem, and smarter than you think.*
>
> **A.A. Milne**

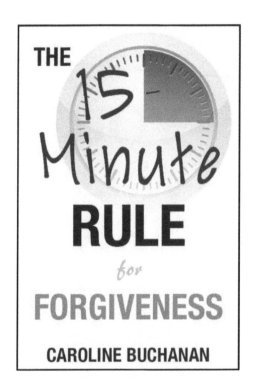

Forgiveness is one of the most powerful and liberating actions a person can take. Whether it is forgiving others, or yourself – for past deeds or mistakes – forgiveness can open people up to a life of happiness, fulfilment, and newfound accomplishment.

The 15-Minute Rule is all about creating a safe framework for fostering forgiveness and self-forgiveness. We can all find 15 minutes in our busy lives and, through the short exercises and examples in the book, forgiveness and mental serenity can be attained.

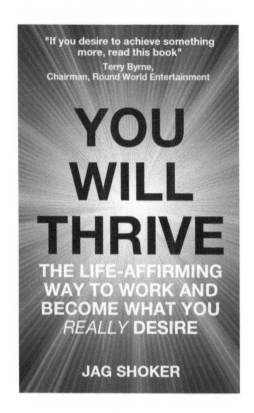

Have you lost your spark or the passion for what you do? Is your heart no longer in your work or (like so many people) are you simply disillusioned by the frantic race to get ahead in life? Your sense of unease may be getting harder to ignore, and comes from the growing urge to step off the treadmill and pursue a more thrilling *and* meaningful direction in life.

You Will Thrive addresses the subject of modern disillusionment. It is essential reading for people looking to make the most of their talents and be something more in life. Something that matters. Something that makes a difference in the world.

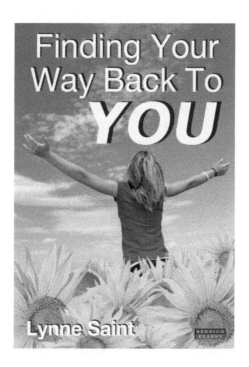

Are you at a crossroads in life, lacking in motivation, looking for a new direction or just plain 'stuck'?

Finding your Way back to YOU is a focused and concise resource written specifically for women who have found themselves in any of the positions above.

The good news is that you already have all of the resources you need to solve your own problems; this practical book helps you remove the barriers that prevent this from happening.

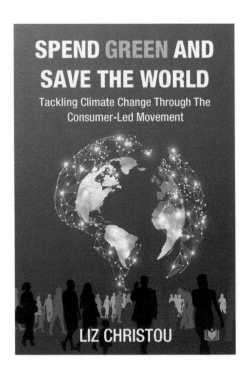

Climate change is the most important issue facing the world today. But are you left wondering what more you can do, personally?

This book is a practical guide on what you can do to make a difference. And the amazing thing is that it only takes 3.5% of a population to act in order to create cultural change, and a mindshift in wider thinking! By coming together and using our consumer power – as part of The Consumer-Led Movement – we can influence businesses and government policy, and rapidly shape a better future. All through consciously choosing how we spend our money.

Other Books from the Publisher

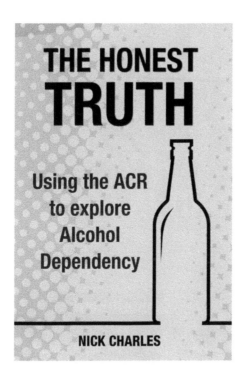

Alcohol dependency – where alcohol has a hold over someone's behaviour – affects people from all walks of life. It can impact an individual's health, wealth, relationships, life fulfilment, and so much more.

In *The Honest Truth*, we explore how to evaluate whether someone has a dependency on alcohol through the ACR: the Alcohol Consumption Regime. It is a focused, simple, six-week programme punctuated with periods of permitted drinking and periods of non-drinking. By the end of it, the reader will see, for themselves, whether alcohol has control over them. With this knowledge in place, they are now better equipped to determine how to move forwards should they need to. The ACR can also be used as a day-to-day routine to moderate and safely control drinking patterns.

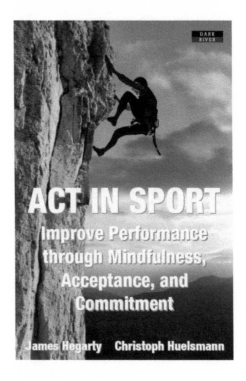

Does unhelpful thinking influence your sporting performance, or the athletes you work with?

Athletes of all levels experience barriers to performance beyond the physical challenges they face. These can range from, performance anxiety, overthinking, and lack of concentration, to issues of motivation or difficulties when dealing with team members. ACT – Acceptance and Commitment Training/Therapy – is a modern and effective psychological approach based on a scientific understanding of human thought and emotional processes. ACT uses a practical and easy-to-use framework for skill development through values-based action, commitment, defusion, mindfulness, and acceptance.